ESSENTIAL FATTY ACIDS
AND TOTAL PARENTERAL NUTRITION
INTERNATIONAL SYMPOSIUM

British Library Cataloguing in Publication Data

Essential fatty acids and total parenteral nutrition.
1. Medicine. Parenteral feeding
I. Ghisolfi, Jacques
615.855

ISBN 0-86196-213-3

Editions John Libbey Eurotext
6, rue Blanche, 92120 Montrouge, France. Tel.: (1)47.35.85.52

John Libbey & Company Ltd
13, Smith Yard, Summerley Street, London SW18 4HR, England
Tel.: (01)947.27.77

John Libbey CIC
Via L. Spallanzani, 11, 00161 Rome, Italy. Tel.: (06)862.289

© John Libbey Eurotext, 1990, Paris

Il est interdit de reproduire intégralement ou partiellement le présent ouvrage – loi du 11 mars 1957 – sans autorisation de l'éditeur ou du Centre Français du Copyright, 6 bis rue Gabriel Laumain, 75010 Paris

ESSENTIAL FATTY ACIDS AND TOTAL PARENTERAL NUTRITION INTERNATIONAL SYMPOSIUM

Proceedings of the International Symposium
April 22-23, 1988, Toulouse, France

Edited by J. Ghisolfi

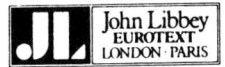

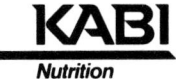

Foreword

This volume contains the proceedings of an International Symposium held in Toulouse in April 22-23, 1988 on essential fatty acids.

This symposium was initiated by Professor Jacques Ghisolfi and Kabi Laboratories were honoured to contribute to the organization of the meeting.

Specialists from several countries gathered to discuss recent development about essential fatty acids. The intention was to bring the audience up to the state of the art in this field.

Kabi involvement in this meeting illustraes the pionneering work of the company in Parenteral Nutrition and the will to support research in this field.

Sincere thanks are due to the speakers and chairmen and to all participants who contributed to the symposium.

A. Kher M.D.
Medical Director
Vice President Kabi France

List of contributors

Adam O., Medizinishe Poliklinik der Universität München Pettenkoferstrafe 8a D-8000 München 2, Federal Republic of Germany

Alcindor L.G., Laboratoire de biochimie, Faculté de médecine de Paris Ouest, 45, rue des Saints Pères, 75006 Paris, France.

Andersen G.E., Department of Neonatalogy, Rigshospitaler, University of Copenhagen, Blegdamsvej 9, DK-21000-Copenhagen, Denmark.

Ane M., Pharmacie, Hôpital Purpan, Place du Docteur Baylac, 31059 Toulouse Cedex, France.

Astre C., C.R.L.C. Clinique St Eloi, 34094 Montpellier, France.

Audigier MJ., Kabivitrum S.A., Le Vendôme, 12-14, rue du Centre, 93167 Noisy le Grand, France.

Bach A., Laboratoire clinique médicale A, Hôpital Civil, 67091 Strasbourg Cedex, France.

Beylot M., INSERM U. 197, Faculté de médecine A. Carrel, rue Guillaume Paradin, 69372 Lyon Cedex 08, France.

Bivins B.A., Henri Ford Hospital, Division of Trauma and critical care surgery, 2799 West Grand Boulevard, Detroit, Michigan 48202, USA.

Bjerve K.S., Department of Clinical Chemistry, Regional Hospital, N-7006 Trondheim, Norway.

Bornet J.L., Service de chirurgie digestive, Hôpital Rangueil, chemin du Vallon, 31054 Toulouse Cedex, France.

Bourre J.M., Unité de neurotoxicologie, INSERM U 26, hôpital Fernand Vidal, 200, rue du Faubourg Saint Denis, 75475 Paris Cedex 10, France.

Bresson, Clinique des maladies des enfants, Hôpital Necker, 149, rue de Sèvres, 75743 Paris Cedex 15, France.

Bunodière M., Kabivitrum S.A., Le Vendôme 12-14, rue du Centre, 93167 Noisy le Grand, France.

Callais F., Laboratoire central de biochimie, Hôpital Laennec, 42, rue de Sèvres, 75007 Paris, France.

Cathala B., Urgences chirurgicales, Hôpital Purpan, place du Docteur Baylac, 31059 Toulouse Cedex, France.

Cary M., Kabivitrum S.A., Le Vendôme 12-14, rue du Centre, 93167 Noisy le Grand, France.

Couvaras O., Service de médecine infantile D, Hôpital Purpan, place du Docteur Baylac, 31059 Toulouse Cedex, France.

Craste de Paulet, Laboratoire de biochimie des lipides, Hôpital Lapeyronie, 555, route de Ganges, 34059 Montpellier Cedex, France.

Cunnane S.C., Department of Nutritional Sciences, Faculty of Medecine, University of Toronto, Toronto, Ontario MSS 1A8, Canada.

Di Costanzo J., Clinique de la Résidence du Parc, Rue Gaston Berger, 13362 Marseille Cedex 10, France.

Doffoel M., Service d'Hépatogastroentérologie, Clinique Médicale B, Hôpital Central, 67091 Strasbourg Cedex, France.

Du Cailar J., Department d'anesthésie réanimation, Hôpital Lapeyronie, 555, route de Ganges, 34059 Montpellier Cedex, France.

Dumont J.C., Département d'anesthésie réanimation, hôpital de la Timone, boulevard Jean Moulin, 13292 Marseille Cedex 6, France.

Ekman L., Kabivitrum Nutrition A.B., S-112 87 Stockholm, Sweden.

Friedman Z., Neonatalogy, 1919 La Branch, Houston, Texas 77002, USA.

Gadrat F., Département d'anesthésie réanimation I, hôpital Pellegrin, 33076 Bordeaux Cedex, France.

Garcia J., Service de médecine infantile D, hôpital Purpan, place du Docteur Baylac, 31059 Toulouse Cedex, France.

Ghisolfi J., Service de médecine infantile D, hôpital Purpan, place du Docteur Baylac, 31059 Toulouse Cedex, France.

Goulet O., Service de Pédiatrie, 149, rue de Sèvres, 75743 Paris Cedex 15, France.

Guillaume O., Kabivitrum S.A., Le Vendôme 12-14, rue du Centre, 93167 Noisy le Grand, France.

Hakansson, Kabivitrum S.A., Z.I.N., rue de Dion Bouton, 87000 Limoges, France.

Hanh T., Kabivitrum S.A., Le Vendôme 12-14, rue du Centre, 93167 Noisy le Grand, France.

Harant Isabelle, Service de médecine infantile D, hôpital Purpan, place du Docteur Baylac, 31059 Toulouse Cedex, France.

Hansen H.S., Denmarks Farmacentiske Hojskole, The Royal Danish School of Pharmacy, Biochemical Laboratory, Universitetsparken 2, DK 2100 Copenhagen, Denmark.

Huang Y.S., Efamol Research Institute, Annapolis Valley Industrial, Park P.O. Box 818, Kentville, Nova Scotia, Canada B 4N 4H8.

Kher A., Kabivitrum S.A., Le Vendôme 12-14, rue du Centre, 93167 Noisy Le Grand, France.

Koletzko B., The Hospital for sick children, Division of Clinical Nutrition, Department of Paediatrics, 555 University Avenue, Toronto, Ontario, Canada MSG 1×8.

Lagarigue F., Hôpital Trousseau, 37044 Chambray les Tours, France.

Leverve X., Service de Réanimation Médicale, Hôpital des Sablons, 38043 Grenoble Cedex, France.

List of contributors

Lindholm M., Kabivitrum Nutrition AB, S-112 87 Stockholm, Sweden.

Lundell S., Kabivitrum Nutrition AB, S-112 87 Stockholm, Sweden.

Mac Lean N., Department of Nutritional Sciences, Faculty of Medecine, University of Toronto, Toronto, Ontario, M 55 1AS, Canada.

Manelli J.C., Department d'anesthésie réanimation, hôpital de la Conception, 144, rue Saint Pierre, 13005 Marseille, France.

Mansini J.P., Département d'anesthésiologie, Hôpital Saint Antoine, 184, rue du Faubourg Saint Antoine, 75571 Paris Cedex 12, France.

Martinez M., Hospital Infantil Vail d'Hebron, Passeig de la Vail d'Hebron, 08035 Barcelona, Spain.

Martins F., Chirurgia Pediatrica, Rua Entro Campos 34, 1700 Lisboa, Portugal.

Menez, Faculté de médecine, Service de biochimie, 22, avenue Camille Desmoulins, B.P. 815, 29285 Brest Cedex, France.

Messing B., Service de gastroentérologie, hôpital Saint Lazare, 107, rue du Faubourg Saint Denis, Paris Cedex 10, France.

Navarro J., Service de pédiatrie, Hôpital Bretonneau, 2, 5 et 7, rue Carpeaux, 75877 Paris Cedex 18, France.

Olives J.P., Service de médecine infantile D, Hôpital Purpan, Place du Docteur Baylac, 31059 Toulouse Cedex, France.

Perrin-Ansart M.C., Kabivitrum S.A., Le Vendôme 12-14, rue du Centre, 93167 Noisy le Grand, France.

Pradere B., Hôpital Purpan, service de chirurgie digestive, place du Docteur Baylac, 31059 Toulouse Cedex, France.

Putet G., Néonatalogie, pavillon J, hôpital Edouard Herriot, 5, place d'Arsonval, 69437 Lyon Cedex 03, France.

Ricour C., Service de pédiatrie, hôpital Necker, 149, rue de Sèvres, 75743 Paris Cedex 15, France.

Rieu D., Service des maladies des enfants, hôpital Saint Charles, 300, rue A. Broussonnet, 34039 Montpellier Cedex, France.

Sami H., C.R.L.C. Cliniques Saint Eloi, 34094 Montpellier, France.

Sanchez R., Service des brûlés, hôpital Pellegrin, place Amélie Raba Léon, 33076 Bordeaux Cedex, France.

Sarda P., Néonatalogie, hôpital Saint Charles, 300, rue A. Broussonnet, 34039 Montpellier Cedex, France.

Saroul Nicole, Kabivitrum S.A., Le Vendôme 12-14, rue du centre, 93167 Noisy le Grand, France.

Sonnenfeld H., Departement d'anesthésie réanimation, hôpital Claude Huriez, place de Verdun, 59037, Lille Cedex, France.

Strub, Service d'anesthésie réanimation, hôpital de Brabois, route de Neufchateau, 54500 Vandœuvre les Nancy, France.

Szawlowski A., C.R.L.C. Clinique Saint Eloi, 34094 Montpellier, France.

Tenenbaum, Service de pédiatrie II, hôpital d'enfants, B.P. 1542, 21034 Dijon Cedex, France.

Thouvenot J.P., Laboratoire central de biochimie II, hôpital Purpan, place du docteur Baylac, 31059 Toulouse Cedex, France.

Voultoury J.C., Service de réanimation, hôpital Dupuytren, avenue Alexis Carel, 87000 Limoges, France.

Wunenburger R., Kabivitrum S.A., Le Vendôme 12-14, rue du centre, 93167 Noisy le Grand, France.

Contents

Foreword V

List of contributors VII

Opening address. *J. Ghisolfi (Toulouse, France), R. Wunenburger (Kabivitrum, France)* XIII

Symposium proceedings

1. Fatty acids and fat emulsions. State of the art. *M. Lindholm (Stockholm, Sweden)* 3
2. The essential nature of linoleic acid in mammals. Linoleic acid and its higher homologues. Which is essential ? *H.S. Hansen (Copenhagen, Denmark)* 15
3. The composition of nerve membranes and enzymatic and electrophysiological (behavioural and toxicological) parameters depend on polyunsaturated fatty acids (especially linolenic acid). Minimum dietary requirements of linoleic and linolenic acids. *J.M. Bourre, O. Dumont, M. Piccioti, G. Pascal, G. Durand (Paris, France)* 23
4. Fatty acid composition of rat tissues during total parenteral nutrition. *(F. Martins, Lisbon, Portugal)* 45
5. Effects of dietary linoleic, and linolenic acids on tissue fatty acids and prostaglandin biosynthesis in animals. *(Y.S. Huang, Kentville, Nova Scottia, Canada)* 51
6. Regulation of essential fatty acid metabolism during total parenteral nutrition. Nutrient interrelations and particularly interactions of zinc and copper. *(S. Cunnane, Toronto, Canada)* 69
7. Linoleic acid intake and prostaglandin formation in man. *(O. Adam, München, West Germany)* 81
8. Essential fatty acids and fat supplemented parenteral nutrition in adult patients. *(B.A. Bivins, Detroit, USA)* 95
9. Metabolic utilization of linoleic acid from fat emulsion during total parenteral nutrition in infants. Fatty acid composition of lipid tissues and prostaglandin synthesis. *(Z. Friedman, Houston, USA)* 111

Essential fatty acids

10. **Which essential fatty acids should be supplied to the newborn infant.** *(B. Koletzko, Toronto, Canada)* 123
11. **Essential fatty acids, parenteral nutrition and the developing human.** *(M. Martinez, Barcelona, Spain)* 139
12. **Does cutaneous application of essential fathy acids (EFA) prevent EFA deficiency during total parenteral nutrition in infants.** *(O. Goulet, C. Ricour, Paris, France)* 151
13. **How to appreciate the adequacy supply of linoleic acid during total parenteral nutrition in clinical practice.** *(J. Ghisolfi, Toulouse, France)* 157
14. **Omega-3 essential fatty acid deficiency and artificial nutrition.** *(K.S. Bjerve, Trondheim, Norway)* 163
15. **New fatty acids in the emulsions of the nineties. Possibilities and limitations.** *(C.M.H. Carneheim, C. Larsson-Backström, L. Ekman Stockholm, Sweden)* 171

This papers correspond either to the tape recorded during the symposium or were totally rewritten by the authors afterwards.

Opening address

Ladies and gentlemen,

You are very welcome to this symposium on Essential Fatty Acids and Total Parenteral Nutrition. It is a pleasure for me to receive you in Toulouse.

More than twenty five years ago, the development of well tolerated fat emulsions made it possible to devise a total parenteral nutrition regimen adequate from a nutritional point of view. This was very important as total parenteral nutrition using hypertonic glucose and aminoacid solutions has led to the recognition of essential fatty acid deficiency state. However prevention and treatment of essential fatty acid deficiency during total parenteral nutrition have not been thoroughly evaluated despite the intensive use of fat emulsion. Now the rapid increase of intravenous fate emulsion during total parenteral nutrition, the increase of our knowledge on fatty acid, on the metabolism of fatty acid during total parenteral nutrition have created the need for a critical appraisal of the state of the art. So, one year ago I thought it might be a good idea to arrange a symposium with the very best specialists in the field of essential fatty acid and total parenteral nutrition.

We are proud and happy to have managed to get almost all those we wanted. Many thanks to all for your collaboration.

Let us now turn to the topics of the symposium. This morning we will speak about fat emulsion, the state of the art and basic knowledge on linoleic and alpha linolenic acids. In the afternoon we will consider some data on fatty acid metabolism and we will begin to consider essential fatty acids in human total parenteral nutrition. Tomorrow morning we will continue to look into this topic and we will finish by considerations on fat emulsions in the future. We have much to learn about how the human body utilizes fatty acid supply parenterally in comparison to those supplied orally. I hope that at the end of this symposium we shall have a better understanding of the problems posed.

J. Ghisolfi

*
* *

Ladies and gentlemen,

R. Wunenburger (Kabivitrum France): Ladies and gentlemen, good morning. Kabivitrum France is happy to welcome you in this splendid and beautiful city of Toulouse and to participate to this symposium organized under the initiative of Prof Ghisolfi, very well known in France for his work on nutrition and especially essential fatty acids. This type of manifestation corresponds exactly to what we like to do and illustrates perfectly what we mean by partnership between university and industry. This exchange of ideas gives the opportunity to make the balance on one aspect of medecine which is making important progress and to exchange points of view which will constitute the therapy of tomorrow.

Opening address

No doubt that the quality of attendees, the fact that a number of nations are represented is only proof of the interest of the subjects which will be studied today and tomorrow. We are sure that these exchanges will be extremely fruitful and will lead to active and positive discussions and now let's start this symposium, thank you.

R. Wunenburger

Prof Ghisolfi: Let us now begin our symposium and it is an honour for me to ask Mr Adam to come to the podium to preside the first session of our meeting.

Dr Adam: So, thank you Prof Ghisolfi and Dr Wunenburger for organizing this marvellous meeting in this lovely town here, I am a little elevated here and I will use this situation just to stick to the schedule of the programme. We will start right now with the first lecture given by Dr Lindholm from Stockholm, Sweden about "Fatty Acids and Fat Emulsion. State of the Art."

Symposium Proceedings

1

Fatty acids and fat emulsions. State of the art

M. LINDHOLM

Kabivitrum Nutrition AB, S-11287 Stockholm, Sweden

M. Lindholm : M. Chairman, ladies and gentlemen, Prof Ghisolfi. I would like to take the opportunity to express my gratitude over the possibility to leave the winter in Sweden for a while and come here to this beautiful city and the spring in the south of France.

The use of fat emulsions adds many advantages to total parenteral nutrition. It offers a high caloric density, provides essential fatty acids and fat soluble vitamins and is isotonic and thus more suitable for peripheral vein administration than hyper osmolar carbohydrates. At similar caloric intake, the dual energy system also has some important metabolic advantages to the fat free regimen. Fat infusion leads to a reduced insulin requirement which is of importance especially in the stressed patient, who often has a poor glucose tolerance due to insulin resistance. In comparison with glucose, fat leads to reduced production of carbon dioxide and a lowered respiratory quotient of importance especially in patients with impaired pulmonary function and or about to be weened off the ventilator. The increased urinary excretion of catecholamines observed in response to high glucose load is not observed when fat containing TPN is given to hyper-metabolic patients. The high incidence of altered liver function tests observed during hyper-caloric administration of glucose is markedly reduced with a mixed regimen.

Exogenous fat particles had been designed to closely resemble endogenous chylomicrons. The size range is similar to the endogenous chylomicrons but the composition markedly differ between endogenous and exogenous lipid particles.

Exogenous triglycerides contain the essential fatty acids, linoleic and linolenic acid. Exogenous particles do not contain cholesterol esters and only very little of free cholesterol. Exogenous particles contain more or less plant sterols which normally is not absorbed from the intestine plant sterols are not easily metabolized in humans but accumulate in the circulation. Phospholipid content varies from one emulsion to another but is always much larger in the exogenous particles than in endogenous chylomicrons. No apolipoproteins are present at exogenous particles while the endogenous particle contains various apolipoproteins.

Essential fatty acids

The metabolism of intravenous fat emulsions resembles that of natural chylomicrons and large VLDL particles with respect to both plasma removal kinetics and interaction with enzyme lipoprotein lipase (*figure 1*). The triglycerides in the exogenous particles are hydrolysed to free fatty acids and glycerol. The fatty acids can be transported through the cell membrane either to adipose tissue where they are resynthesized into triglycerides for storage or to the muscle for betaoxidation to energy. In addition an appreciable amount of released free fatty acids are bond to albumin and recirculate causing an increase in plasma free fatty acid concentration which is also readily used as fuel. In the liver, curculating free fatty acids may be converted into VLDL and resecreted into plasma. Lipoprotein lipase is the key enzyme in the hydrolysis of triglyceride-rich particles. The hydrolysis by lipoprotein lipase in capillaries of adipose tissue is the step that determines the rate at which fatty acids from lipoproteins are transported into the tissue for storage. Unlike many other key enzymes, lipoprotein lipase can be regulated both in amount and in activity. The amount of active lipoprotein lipase at the capillary endothelium is under hormonal control. Apoliproprotein C2 is a specific activator of lipoprotein lipase and the enzyme is virtually inactive in the absence of its activator.

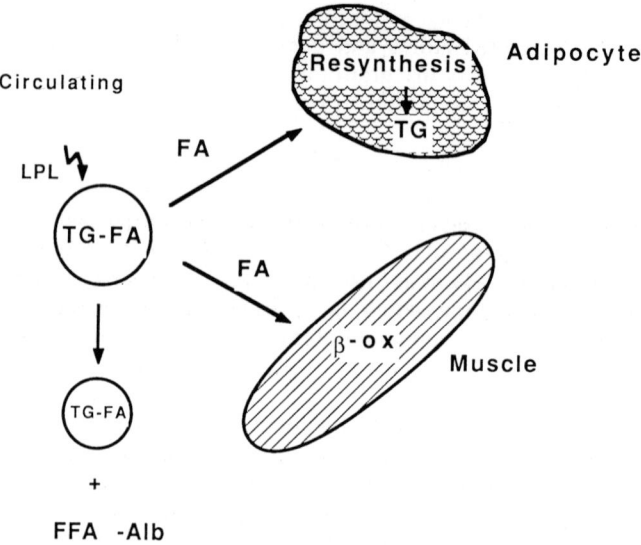

Figure 1. Fatty acid metabolism.

Fatty acids are classified into three main families, omega 3, 6 and 9 characterized by the length of the carbon chain, number of double bonds and position of the double bonds (*figure 2*). Fatty acids are elongated and desaturated at the carboxylic end, thus maintaining their omega family during synthesis of new fatty acid compound. Whereas those omega 3 and 6 fatty acid family members can be synthesized in the body the parent fatty acids, linoleic and linolenic acids, cannot and must therefore be supplied. The polyunsaturated fatty acids are biosynthetic precursors to prostaglandins, thromboxanes and leukotrienes. Infusion of fat emulsions may

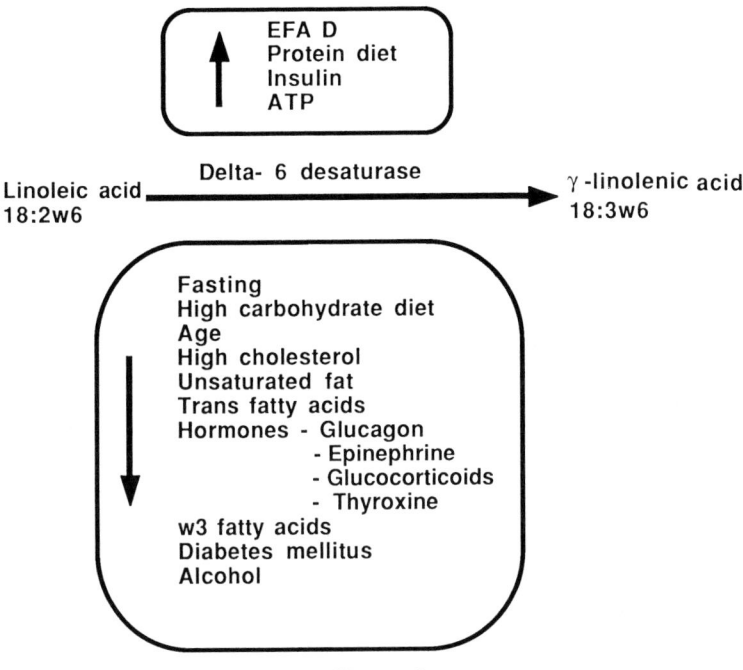

Figure 2

have profound physiologic and pharmacologic actions aside from provision of calories. These effects may be beneficial for patients suffering from pulmonary diseases, cystic fibrosis etc. Alterations in the prostaglandin production occur dependent on the fatty acid profile of the dietary oil fat or intravenous fat emulsion given. Delta 6 desaturase is the rate limiting enzyme for metabolism of both omega 3 and omega 6 fatty acids. The omega 3 and omega 6 fatty acids compete with each other for both storage in phospholipids as part of the membranes and for transformation to prostaglandins and leukotrienes and this is the so-called polyenoic competition. Omega 3 fatty acids and their metabolites have competitive and inhibitory effects on the metabolism of linoleic acid. An absolute or relative excess of linolenic acid intake results in an abnormal fatty acid metabolite profile and of abnormal membrane structures. Most of the abnormalities following excessive linolenic acid intake can be ascribed to preferential incorporation of omega 3 fatty acids into the membrane phospholipids. Red blood cell abnormal shape and fragility, anaemia, altered platelet aggregation and impaired cellular respiratory capacity secondary to changes in mitochondrial architecture are only a few findings in animals and humans fed soybean, linseed or fish oils for periods varying between 30 and 300 days. Only 1.1% of calories as linolenic acid are required to induce a 50% inhibition of the conversion of linoleic acid to $22:5\omega6$. However a certain amount of linolenic acid must be supplied in order to prevent essential fatty acid deficiency. I think we will hear a lot more about this during these two days.

One of the advantages with fat emulsions is the possibility to supply essential fatty acids. Holman found that the ratio between trienoic and tetraenoic 20:3 to

20:4 acids, can be used as an expression of essential fatty acid deficiency, a value of 4 or greater defining essential fatty acid deficiency.

A supply of linoleic acid is important for normal synthesis of arachidonic acid. It is a stepwise conversion of linoleic acid over gammalinolenic acid, dihomogammalinolenic acid to arachidonic acid. The enzyme delta 6 desaturase is a rate limiting enzyme. The activity of the delta 6 desaturase can be influence by a number of clinical conditions and therapies. The enzyme activity is increased by essential free fatty acid deficiency, aminoacid intake, insulin etc., while fasting, high carbohydrate diet, age and several other clinical conditions decrease the delta 6 desaturase acivity.

There are three main functions of essential fatty acids, the most important is as part of phospholipids in all animal cellular membranes. In deficiency of essential fatty acids faulty membranes are formed. Secondly, essential fatty acids act as precursors of prostanoids which are only formed from essential fatty acids and the last function is, of course, as energy source.

EFA deficiency has been described in infants on prolonged fat free parenteral nutrition and the clinical findings include dermatitis, thrombocytopenia, increased susceptibility to bacterial infections and failure to thrive. During pregnancy and inpremature infants the minimum requirement of essential fatty acids is about 1% of energy. More optimal is to give about 4% of the non protein energy as essential fatty acids. A deficiency in these groups are associated with retarded growth, reduced maturation and irreversible central nervous system damage. Other clinical conditions at risk for developing a functional essential fatty acid deficiency are patients with burns, trauma and alcoholics.

There seems to be an optimal ratio between linoleic and linolenic acid intake. The fatty acid pattern of human breast milk might be considered as an adequate guideline particular in infants. The ratio linoleic to linolenic acid in breast milk is about 7 to 13 and it varies with the diet of the mother. In intralipid it is about 7 while in the safflower containing fat emulsion (Liposyn) it is significantly higher. Adult animals tend to incorporate both fatty acids (linoleic and linolenic acids) in their membranes in the proportion 1:1 to 5:1. The fatty acid composition of different fat emulsions is thus of great interest. For example eicosapentanoic acid is decreased during infusion of safflower oil containing fat emulsions while it is increased when soybean emulsions are given.

In a comparative study in adults, Cook and co-workers noted higher plasma triglyceride concentrations and a decreased clearance during safflower oil infusion compared with soybean oil (*Table I*).

Table I. Plasma triglycerides during safflower oil and soybean oil infusion (Cook *et al.*, 1983)

	n	Hour			
		0	2	4	8
Safflower oil(mg/dl)	18	58 ± 29	156 ± 56	195 ± 91	208 ± 95
Soybean oil(mg/dl)	18	53 ± 25	133 ± 39	153 ± 42	162 ± 85
P		NS	< 0.05	< 0.001	< 0.001

Data expressed as mean ± SD.
NS. Not significant.

Hailer and Wolfram in Munich have compared Lipofundin and Intralipid, two soybean based fat emulsions. Lipofundin was faster eliminated from the circulation than Intralipid. In premature infants however there was no difference. The major difference in composition between these two emulsions are the emulsifier and the content of cholesterol.

In the area of parenteral nutrition we have been limited for many years to lipid emulsions based on soybean or safflower oil. Both are long chaine triglycerides (LCT) types. Medium chain triglycerides (MCT)fat emulsions have been in clinical use for some years but the potential pros and cons are still frequently discussed. MCT emulsion contains C6 – C12 fatty acids and the fatty acid distribution in LCT fat emulsion and MCT is shown on *Table II*. And as you can see for the considered emulsion 65% – 75% of fatty acid contents in MCT emulsions is caprillic acid, C8. MCT demonstrates certain additional characteristics of some advantage whereas LCT generally are slowly metabolized to energy or stored. MCT are metabolized as rapidly and completely as glucose and having twice the caloric density of protein and carbohydrates. The oxidation of MCT are not dependent on carnitine in contrast to the oxidation of LCT, at least not completely. LCT on the other hand are dependent on carnitine for the transport over the inner mitochondrial membrane. MCT are easily oxidized and utilized for energy with only a little tendency to deposit in the liver or adipose tissue. Since MCT readily undergo beta-oxidation ketonemia is usually much more pronounced than with LCT emulsions. Skeletal muscle can easily burn ketone bodies for energy and may thus spare the oxidation of branched chain amino-acids and reduce skeletal protein catabolism. However the development of MCT emulsions has been hampered by the fact that a tolerence has been low. It was demonstrated that triglycerides with shorter fatty acid chain lengths had pronounced toxic effects. The negative effects are increased thermogenesis as a result of an

Table II. Fatty acid composition of the lipid emulsions* (Granger *et al.*, 1987)

	Fatty acids	%
LCT emulsion	C16:0	12.03
	C18:0	4.51
	C18:1	23.28
	C18:2	53.42
	C18:3	7.60
	C20:4	0.00
MCT emulsion	C6:0	0.18
	C8:0	65.85
	C10:0	30.34
	C12:0	1.03
	C14:0	0.12
	C16:0	1.84
	C18:0	0.73
	C20:4	0.00

* The levels are expressed as percentages of total fatty acid content. It is important to remember that the LCTs were infused as such, whereas the MCTs were infused after vol/vol dilution with LCTs

increased energy expenditure, risk for metabolic acidosis and enlarged doses MCT might cause meurotoxic symptoms, for example coma. MCT also suffer from the absence of EFAs, patients who get MCT containing fat emulsions also gain less body weight than LCT emulsions.

During an infusion of MCT/LCT mixture, the plasma level of arachidonic acid was significantly higher and the C18 level lower than during the LCT treatment. It's arachidonic acid at the top. This supports the hypothesis that MCT/LCT infusion enhances the elongation and the desaturation of 18:2 to 20:4. As MCT are preferentially used as energy and simultaneously infused, essential fatty acids becomes more available for elongation and desaturations. When only LCT are infused part of the long chain fatty acids have to be used as fuel supply and cannot be elongated with the same efficiency.

During TPN there is also an immediate increase of plasma triglyceride concentration, this increase is much faster with LCT than with MCT/LCT. Only 30% of LCT is directly oxidized when given intravenously in fat emulsions and this is similar to what is seen when fat is part of normal diet. The rest of the triglycerides are taken up by the various tissues and utilized later. MCT on the other hand is more directly oxidized. In a study by Prof. Ekhard and his group the oxidation rate of MCT was studied using indirect calosimetry (*figure 3*). The MCT part is oxidized during the eight hours infusion at a cost of an increased oxygen consumption. LCT on the other hand is utilized slower but as complete over 24h.

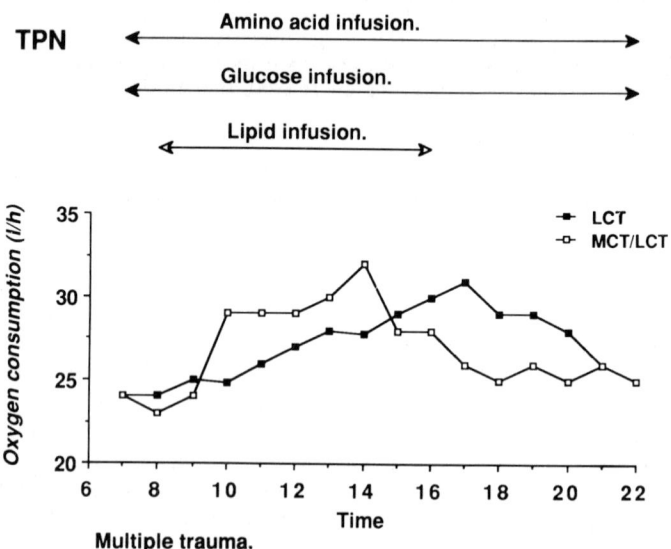

Figure 3. Oxidation rate of MCT using indirect calosimetry (*Eckart et al. 1986*).

It is not only the fatty acid composition of fat emulsions that is important for the different effects of intravenous fat emulsions. The rate of infusion is important, a slow infusion of fat results in a relative predominance of vasodilating prostaglandin E substances while a rapid infusion overwhelms this pathway and leads to predominance vasoconstrictive in prostaglandins. The vasodilating effects of PGE PGI2 have been used clinically to treat pulmonary hypertension and improve blood flow in peripheral vascular disease and for maintaining patency of ductus arteriosus in newborns. The effects of intravenous fat emulsions appear also to be dependent on the duration of the infusion, 2h to 4h infusion time seems to be too short for an anti-inflammatory response, 12h infusion in patients whith cystic fibrosis results on the other hand in an anti-inflammatory and pulmonary response. It is also important whether the emulsion is given as a cyclic or continuous infusion and in a study by our organiser Prof Ghisolfi and co-workers it was shown that the continuous infusion resulted in higher concentrations of linoleic acid and its metabolites, and that cyclic infusion indicated a better essential fatty acid status than a continuous infusion.

I would now like to sum up showing two slides: Holman stated the importance of providing EFAs to patients on TPN (*figure 4*). It cannot be justified not to give

> "EFA-deficiency has been unknowinlgy induced in countless humans by the life saving use of total parenteral nutrition without EFA. Now that this has been amply demonstrated , the continued use of preparations without fat emulsions cannot be justified. The composition of such emulsions and the dosage should be tuned more closely to provide for the full requirement of both families of essential PUFA".
>
> R. Holman 1987

Figure 4

fat emulsions in the TPN programme. The composition of the emulsion, the way of administration are also important factors for the effect of a fat emulsion. Fat emulsions used, should be thought of not only as a caloric source and a source for EFAs but it might be possible to use intravenous fat emulsions as pharmacologic agents to achieve prostaglandin related anti-inflammatory response, anti-platelet aggregation and changes in membrane function and vaso-motor tone and to correct errors in prostaglandin synthesis. Considering the theoretical possibilities intravenous fat emulsions offer an exciting future of which we will hear much more during this meeting. Thank you.

Summary

The use of fat emulsions adds many advantages to TPN: it offers a high caloric density, provides essential fatty acids and fat soluble vitamins, and is isotonic and hence suitable for peripheral vein administration. Metabolism of intravenous fat emulsions (IVFE) is similar to that of endogenous chylomicrons with respect to both plasma removal kinetics and interaction with lipoprotein lipase. The triglycerides (TG) in chylomicrons are hydrolyzed to free fatty acids (FFA) and glycerol. The FA are transported in plasma bound to albumin and are either used for energy or stored in adipose tissue.

FA are characterized by their length, number of double bonds and position of double bonds. FA of different w-families are uniformly distributed in naturally occuring oils. Dietary ingestion favouring one type of oil over another will lead to different FA profiles in the tissues. Absence of w-6 FA acids inthe diet is known as essential fatty acid deficiency and may be corrected by adding linoleic acid and arachinodic acid.

Todays IVFE consists to a great extent of polyunsaturated FA (PUFA) which serve as precursors to prostaglandin synthesis. It may be possible to use IVFE as a pharmacologic agent to achieve prostaglandin related anti-inflammatory and vasomotor tone responses as well as to correct errors in prostaglandin synthesis. The rate and duration of the infusion of IVFE is also of importance for the prostaglandin response.

Fatty acids are also important energy substrates. The long chain FA need carnitine to be transported into the mitochondria where the beta-oxidation takes place.

Medium chain fatty acids, on the other hand, are only partly carnitine dependent for their oxidation and are more rapidly oxidized than long chain FA. Medium chain FA are an interesting alternative especially in the critically ill patient with a high energy need. There are however some disadvantages with the use of medium chain FA.

Todays IVFE are in general well tolerated and frequently used as a caloric source. By modulating the content of PUFA, FA pattern, infusion rate etc it may be possible to use the pharmacologic effects of IVFE by influencing the inflammatory respons and other prostaglandin mediated effects on vasomotor tone and platelet aggregation.

Discussion

Dr Adam: Thank you Dr Lindholm for your marvellous speech and putting all those things into an order about fat infusions and I really want to take the opportunity to ask you for questions. There's a lot to ask about that, many of the points we will hear about this afternoon.

Dr Bjerve: What about the possibilitiy of developing or increasing the risk of developing EFA deficiency when you include high amounts of medium chain triglycerides in the diet. There have been some reports indicating that MCTs well increase the need of supplying EFAs. What is your opinion?

M. Lindholm: I have no personal experience with MCTs since it's not available in Sweden yet, but what I've seen in the literature I agre that there is an increased risk of increasing essential fatty acid deficiency if you give too much of it. So I think that it's essential that you have a good balance between long chain and MCT fatty acids, but I've no personal experience.

Prof Ghisolfi: You said there is a very good ratio between omega 6 and omega 3 fatty acids in intralipid; how do you find this ratio more than 25 years ago? On what concept?

M. Lindholm: That maybe we can ask Dr. Hakanson who is here because I was not participating in that development.

Dr Hakanson: We didn't discuss this problem at that time, 1960, when intralipid was born, I think we had a lot of work to prepare an emulsion with nontoxic effects; so we didn't know anything about this problem.

M. Lindholm: So I think we were just lucky.

Dr Cunnane: I think it's interesting to look at the fatty acid percentage in intralipid and in human milk giving a ratio of omega 3 to omega 6, because although the linoleic/linolenic ratio in milk is possibly 12 or 13 as you say, the total omega 6 to total omega 3 ratio is not that; it's closer to 4 to 5 maybe 6 and I think that's a more realistic measure of the importance of the two families rather than a 12 to 1 ratio.

M. Lindholm: I agree.

Prof Bivins: We can go back to the MCT question for just a moment, I've looked at a blend of 45% MCT v 55% LCT and did not see a change in the ratio of the longer homologues that are synthesized, most of that problem came with the 75% MCT infusions that were used originally for research purposes, the same with the neurologic symptoms they are much less as youcome down closer toa 50 – 50 split.

M. Lindholm: And it's also much lower if you combine it with glucose which should be remembered and that's the normal way to administer; it as part of a TPN program.

Essential fatty acids

Dr Messing: Concerning your comparison between glucose and fat delivery during TPN, about liver function test, I think it's better to compare such regimen when essential fatty acid is covered because it's essential need for the body. So I am asking you what about the liver function test when you give either essential fatty acid dose to prevent or correct EFA deficiency status plus energy source or glucose versus lipid (50/50) for example?

M. Lindholm: There are studies from a group in England, Hall. Burgess and co-workers where they looked upon in a comparative study fat free diet, not providing essential free fatty acids and only glucose, but they did it in the very early period, the first week of TPN and during that time, essential fatty acid should not develop if the patient is not in a very hyperdynamic state, and they could see that the anti pyrine clearance as a measure of liver function was significantly decreased indicating that the enzyme P4 50 system was really very low if you give only glucose; but when you added fat, 30% – 40% fat, it was normalized within a couple of days. That's the only study I know that they've looked very, very early during TPN when fatty acid deficiency is not likely to have occured yet.

Prof Bach: May I come back on MCT. I think it's important to say that MCT are never infused alone; that is a very important point; they are always infused with long chain triglycerides. So you have no deficiency in essential fatty acids. Another point you have no acidosis because you infuse long chain triglycerides in the same time and I think the increase in ketodemia is very slow; you infuse always glucose in the same time so the increase in ketone bodies is very small.

M. Lindholm: Yes, but you should infuse glucose in parrallel.

Prof Bach: May I tell what I heard in Las Vegas at the Aspen meeting. It has been told that one of the interests of medium chain triglycerides may be that its supply of medium chain triblycerides may reduce the supply of long chain triglycerides and thus it would be decrease some problems which coulc arise with long chain triglycerides and which supply of too much long chain essential fatty acids.

M. Lindholm: But I still think we have really to look upon what implication the mixture had on prostaglandin metabolism so that we can manipulate that in the way we want to.

Chairman: So it's very important issue and we should really give way for one further question and then move on to our next paper.

Dr Koletzko: I would like to put a small question mark besides your beautiful slide on the definition of essential acid deficiency. You cited Dr Holman who proposed, I guess, in his early studies in rats and further on in infants that the triene tetraene ratio larger than .4 would be the criterion for EFA deficiency. I believe that in a later report of the FAO in Rome there was agreement that this ratio should be lowered 0:2 as a criterion for EFA deficiency. But also I think it is very important to differentiate where you measure that people have used; this as a very strict criterion and if you look at the different lipid fraction of plasma total lipids the normal range is very different. The other point is that as you have demonstrated clearly in your beautiful slides the triene/tetraene ratio depends on the competition between linoleic plus alphalinolenic and oleic acid so, on the concentrations on these three fatty acids and also on the activity of the desaturating and chain elongating enzyme system and first of all we know that in human the activity of this enzyme system is probably lower than in the experimental rats in which the whole idea was developed and also in many of our patients the activity may be further reduced; for example we have found that in children with malnutrition the delta 6 desaturase activity is very low so they will not develop a high triene/tetraene ratio even if they are essential fatty acid deficient or the same may be true for the newborn infant or the premature infant.

M. Lindholm: And the elderly patient: that's very true and I could not include everything.

Chairman: But you included quite a lot and we thank you once more for your nice lecture and we really should move on to Dr Hansen from Copenhagen, Denmark giving us a lecture about "The essential nature of linoleic acid in mammals."

2

The essential nature of linoleic acid in mammals. Linoleic acid and its higher homologues. Which is essential?

H.S. HANSEN

Biochemical laboratory, Danmarks Farmaceutiske Mojskobe, The Royal Danish School of Pharmacy, Universitetsparken 2, DK-2100 Copenhagen, DenmarK

Dr Hansen: I'm a biochemist and not a clinician and I'll be talking about the essential fatty acids and animal studies and the more principal discussion of why, how they are essential.

This is how it all began. In the 1920s when people were studying vitamin deficiency and working on tocopherol, vitamin E and they wanted to produce an assay using a rat which was given a fat free diet and then discovered fat deficiency symptoms and fat deficiency which was found to be cured by linoleic acid; this is how such an EFA deficient rat looks like. What you can't see here is that it's smaller than the control rat, it is scaly skin on the tail, on the feet, dandruff, it loses its hair and it drinks the double of water as the control rat. A normal rat drinks about 20 – 25 ml/day, this one will drink 45 ml/day, and still it is smaller and sometimes it excretes less urine than the control rat.

Considering the growth curb, the body weight curb, of three groups of rats all fed the same fat free diet, one group being fed fat free diet, the second group being fed with a fat free diet supplemented with linoleic acid. The third group is fed fat free diet supplemented with alphalinolenic acid we can see that linoleic acid increases the growth rate and it will continue whereas it will stop in the fat free diet in the EFA deficient rats. Alphalinolenic acid has an effect of its own in increasing the growth. If you look at the triene/tetraene ratio in these animals it will be high in the EFA deficient rats. These rats are also linoleic acid deficient; they look just the same, they have scaly skin, they have hair loss, they have decreased growth, they have increased water evaporation but the triene/tetraene ratio is the same as in the one giving linoleic acid; that's because alphalinolenic acid influence the triene/tetraene ratio.

These are the classical symptoms described by. Burr and Burr of EFA deficiency, these are pathological, that is disease symptoms, that is impairment of growth and weight gain, scaly skin, loss of hair, dandruff, increased water consumption. It has later been shown that this increased water consumption is due to increased loss of water over the skin, that is an ineffective water permeability barrier in skin. Impairment of reproductive function and sterility, and kindney degeneration and one further is increased susceptibility to bacteria that means that is an ineffective immune system.

These are the disease symptoms; I have not included the triene tetraene ratio because it's a biochemical index, it does not say there is a deficiency is actually; it just says it's a change in metabolism of fatty acids.

This, originally it was found in the rat and for several years people said this never happened inhumans; then by giving TPN it was found that dermatitis could occur in human beings very rapidly when fat was not used, giving evidence of development of EFA deficiency status.

Let us now rapidly look at linoleic acid metabolism. Some part of linoleic acid ingested is oxidized. Another part of linoleic acid is then desaturated and converted and elongated to the other fatty acids. Arachidonic acid with 20 carbon atoms and 4 double bonds is the one whose accumulating in the phospholipids of cell membranes, whereas the other fatty acids is not very often found in tissues. Arachidonic acid is precursor for prostaglandins, leukotrienes with 4 double bonds, just as dihomogammalinolenic acid is precursor for the monoene prostaglandins. This have probably no normal physiological relevance because there's nearly no dihomogammalinolenic acid in tissues. Some exceptions are the kidney and the seminal vesicles which has high levels of dihomogammalinolenic acid. Considering the metabolism of the n − 9 family oleic acid, normally oleic acid is not elongated and desaturated, only when alphalinolenic acid and linoleic acid is not present in the diet.

Another family of fatty acids, n − 7 fatty acids, also accumulate in EFA deficiency these are the palmitoleic fatty acid family. One of these fatty acids is the 20;4n − 7 fatty acids. Actually it's very difficult to seperate arachidonic acid and 20:4n − 7 on gas chromatography In EFA deficient rats as a shoulder on the peak of arachidonic acid and this can, depending on which tissue you're looking at be up to 50% of the arachidonic acid peak; so you should be careful of saying whether it actually are arachidonic acid or whether it's 20:4n − 7.

These are the possible specific function of the n − 6 fatty acids, what are they doing in the bottom. Everybody say that they are important for proper function of cell membranes. In the 70s, Holman stated that every cell membrane must have arachidonic acid or otherwise it would be faulty and the cell would collapse or something like that. Surely they are precursor for the eicosanoids. They are also precursor for other oxygenated metabolites. We will in the coming year see further studies about biological effects of linoleic acid derivatives. There is a 13 hydroxy octadecanoic acid which has been found and which has biological activity. Then there seems to be a specific function in lipids in the epidermal permeability barrier and then cholesterol transport, arachidonic acids are found in cholesterol esters and have something to do with transport of cholesterol.

This probably has nothing to do with the EFA deficiency symptoms, so I will not discuss this further but I'll take these four points one by one.

Are the n − 6 fatty acids essential for normal function of membranes in general, what I mean is in general is that for all the types is it important? And the evidence against this is that you can have cell cultures without any n − 6 fatty acids, they grow, they divide, they are well functioning; everything seems to be OK in these cell cultures. They produce themselves oleic acid and incorporate oleic acid in cell membranes. They produce an unusual phospholipid containing two oleic acids, but they seem to be able to function just as a celle having linoleic acid. Some cells require for better growth linoleic acid and what they do is they convert linoleic acid to arachidonic acid, and convert arachidonic acid to prostaglandins and prostaglandins are used as growth factors. The other point is there is no specificity converning the term membrane fluidity. Any unsaturated fatty acid seems to function just as well as arachidonic acid will do in terms of melting point and in terms of specificity for membrane enzymes. Of course there are some membrane enzymes which are influenced but it is not the general phenomenon. You cannot just say that if you decrease the n − 6 fatty acids in membrane the enzymes will not function, some will not, some will do, and you cannot say from one cell type to the other. So I think the evidence for this is very poor. They are essential for some cell membranes.

Can eicosanoid formation explain the essential nature of n − 6 fatty acids? The evidence against this is if you give aspirin, aspirin can inhibit prostaglandin formation very efficiently and you do not see EFA deficiency in the symptons from aspirin. That of course does only explain the prostaglandin part of the eicosanoids.

Then there's colombinic acid, colombinic acid is a fatty acid isolated from the seed of the plant colombine; it's quite unusual; it has 18 carbon atom, 3 double bonds and 2 of the double bonds are equivalent to those found in linoleic acid and they have further 5 trans double bond. This fatty acid cannot be elongated and desaturated within the organism. But still it has activity as a EFA, it can cure the classical deficiency symptoms in the rat. Increased growth and decreased transepidermal water loss; there is something it probably can't do; it probably can't cure the fertility deficiency symptoms and probably can't cure the immune deficiency symptoms. And then, there's dietary studies with the cat. The cat has so low delta 6 desaturase that it practically can't convert linoleic acid to arachidonic acid and if you have EFA deficient cats and feed them linoleic acid the deficiency symptoms are cured without they are converting linoleic acid to arachidonic acid. Most of the deficiency symptoms are cured.

Let us now see the relation between skin and essential fatty acids. In the cell membrane there are bodies which has lipid stacks; these stacks seems to be excreted from cell forming lamilla layers of lipid between the cells, and these probably are forming the water barrier of the skin. They are composed of cholesterol esters and ceramides and some of the ceramides are quite unusual in that they are having linoleic acid bound to the ceramides. Linoleic acid rich-lipids, such as acylglucosylceramide, acylceramide and acyl acid have been identified in the epidermis of humans. In EFA deficient rats, the linoleic acid of these epidermal sphingolipids is replace by oleic acid, a replacement which is associated with a loss of barrier function. Apparently acylglucosylceramide is formed in the lamella bodies of the cells and after secretion converted to acylceramide and acyl acid which in some way takes part in the formation of the water permeability barrier. That seems to be why linoleic acid is important for the formation of the barrier. I would say one thing that EFA deficient rats have increased water loss but you cannot compare that by rats with loss at total epidermis then the water loss would be much higher. The water barrier is still functioning without linoleic acid, it's just not as efficient as if linoleic acid is present.

So I would conclude that linoleic acid appears to be an essential fatty acid in its own right for the epidermal permeability barrier that is linoleic acid does not have to be transformed to arachidonic acid. Arachidonic acid may be important for parturition and for proper function of blood platelets and the immune system and this probably is because all of these I mentioned here prostaglandins are important for proper function. Prostaglandins are involved in the parturition, prostaglandins are involved in platelets, and leukotrienes are involved in the immune system. So these are all seen as deficiency symptoms in EFA deficient rats and these symptoms may be correlated with arachidonic acid and eicosanoids. Thank you.

Summary

For more than 50 years ago, Burr & Burr described a dietary fat deficiency syndrome in young rats. They coinced the terme "essential fatty acid" to include all fatty acids, that when included in the diet in a utilizable form, prevent or ameliorate the deficiency disease. All the (n − 6)-fatty acids, linoleic acid, Y-linolenic acid, dihomo-Y-linolenic acid and arachidonic acid, have curative effects on the deficiency symptoms in rats raised on fat-free diet. The term "essential fatty acid" is related to a fatty acid in the diet, and in practice it is linoleic acid, which is the essential nutrient because this acid is the most abundant dietary (n − 6)-fatty. However, which fatty acid(s) is/are the essential metabolite(s)? A part of the dietary linoleate is converted to arachidonic acid in the organism. Arachidonate is relative to other (n − 6)-fatty acids found in high amounts in membrane phospholipids, and arachidonic acid is precursor for the biological active eicosanoids. On this background many nutritionist have suggested that arachidonic acid is the essential metabolite. However, results obtained within the recent years have pointed to linoleic acid as an essential metabolite, having effect without being converted to arachidonic acid. Linoleic acid seems to be essential for the integrity of the epidermal water permeability barrier, a function which indirectly may be important for growth and energy utilization of young animals. Arachidonic acid may be important for proper eicosanoid formation, and thereby affecting such diverse physiological processes as parturition, platelet aggregation and immune response.

Discussion

Dr Adam: Thank you Dr Hansen for your really critical paper and I think there's a lot of things which need to be discussed in your paper, we ask for the first questions please.

Dr Ekman: I have not a question but a comment, since you asked whether there was anyone who had an experience or knew of studies where you studied EFA deficiency in the paediatric situation and where you could prove that there was a water loss. Just before going here, I spoke of this issue with Prof Wretlind; indeed there are such studies and they have shown indirectly by measuring energy expenditure in EFA deficient neonates as compared to normal neonates, and the energy expenditure is about 70% higher; there's an indirect measurement of the water loss to maintain the normal temperature.

Dr Hansen: But it is very important to compare the neonates from the same day because the water permeability barrier is formed around the birth. That is premature infants have a very high water loss, and it's rapidly decreasing after maturation, after the birth of the premature infants; so it's very critical to compare the exact age of the premature infant.

Dr Cunnane: We talk about essential fatty acid deficient infant with some dermatitis, with lots of subcutaneous fat which presumably contains some linoleic acid. Is there any explanation for how the deficiency appears to develop at the skin when right below literally mm away in adiposites we have presumably some linoleic acid.

Dr Hansen: The explanation I have seen in the literature says that it's due to insulin of the high carbohydrate infusions which leads to that you can't mobilize fatty acid from fat tissue, and that should be the reason.

Chairman: Let us stick just for a moment to these symptoms of linoleic acid deficiency in man and I would like to ask if anybody has some experience with linoleic acid deficient symptoms in children or in adults, especially I should like to ask the question whether there is some experience with a functional EFA deficiency?

Dr Koletzko: In fact there is a very old report published who described the same failure to thrive that you just demonstrated in rats, in EFA deficiency in infants.

Prof Friedman: Is there other losses than loss of water during essential fatty acid deficiency status?

Dr Hansen: Yes, because the water barrier is also a barrier to other substances and for instance when the defect water barrier was discovered, Hugh Sinclair was one of the first to describe the defect water barrier. He could put the rats into water and then they accumulated water, the water went in the other way or he tried to get rid of the hair and he put some chemical on the skin and it was actually toxic because the chemical went into the skin, so the skin is open for other things than water.

Dr Messing: I understand what you said about the skin, but for tissues who are growing very fast, for example GI tract and epidelium from the intestine, did you observe any abnormalities in the gut such as diarrhoea or modified permeability, modified transport of sodium and so on?

Dr Hansen: I have not looked at that.

Chairman: So actually it's very difficult to estimate the need for EFAs in animals or anywhere because an organism suffering from EFA deficiency always is under condition where you, it's hard to evaluate the effect of those fatty acids and I think we should just move a little bit on, no I don't want to dismiss you yet, to your question concerning the essentiallity of linoleic acid in cell cultures. There have been a lot of reports indicating that tumors being grown with linoleic acid showing some inhibition of tumor growth with linolenic acid and this growth of tumor was related to the effect of a linoleic acid deficiency. Would you comment a little bit on that?

Dr Hansen: I have seen some of the literature on that and I feel confused. Of course somebody's saying having an effect and I seen also someone saying it's not so good an effect, so I think I wouldn't comment on that now.

Chairman: It certainly depends on the amount of linolenic acid which is present in the medium and that's what I wanted to ask. Don't you think the result from the cell culture studies are a little bit spectacular.

Dr Hansen: Yes, the cell cultures are abnormal in that the cells do not need to communicate and they have an optimal function and they are not stressed. They have all what they need and then they grow of course and that is a drawback of cell cultures surely. But I used only the cell cultures as a point for, that can exist cells which apparently do not need linoleic acid and I've also seen some papers about organisms which may exist without linoleic acid, that's the banana fly. People has raised banana flies on diet totally devoid of linoleic acid.

Chairman: So banana flies don't need intralipid!

Dr Hansen: They form and they don't produce it, some insects produce linoleic acid but they do not.

Chairman: So another point is that aspirin in humans does not inhibit prostaglandin production totally, there's always a raised prostaglandin production of about 30% which cannot be inhibited by aspirin or anything else, so the point is that you can't compare the cell culture results with human studies.

Dr Hansen: No, this was just several different point which I hoped would together form evidence.

Dr Cunnane: Just in relation to this point about aspirin though, Prof Galli, about ten years ago presented a case of a child who was apparently devoid of cyclo-oxygenase activity; do you agree that that case was in fact devoid of cyclo-oxygenase activity indicating a minimal requirement for prostaglandin synthesis?

Dr Hansen: Yes there's been a report in Sweden on the same and one from Japan also about, but I don't know how reliable they are.

Chairman: There was no follow-up report and the report was very incomplete. So thank you once more for your nice lecture and we will move on to Mr Bourre coming from Paris and giving us a lecture about the long title "The composition of nerve membranes and enzymatic and electrophysiological behaviour and toxilogical parameters depend on polyunsaturated fatty acids.

3

Minimum linolenic acid, and linoleic acid requirement for developing brain and various organs.
Fatty acid composition of nervous membranes, control of enzymatic activity, amplitude of electrophysiological parameters, resistance to poisons, and performance of learning tasks[1]

J. BOURRE, O. DUMONT, M. PICIOTTI, G. PASCAL, G. DURAND*

INSERM U 26, Hôpital Fernand Widal, 200 rue du faubourg St-Denis, 75475 Paris Cedex 10, France
*INRA-CNRZ, 78350 Jouy-en-Josas, France

Introduction

The dietary importance of polyunsaturated fatty acids is well known. These compounds contribute to the decreased incidence of cardiovascular disorders, and they are the precursors of biologically active derivatives. Nevertheless, the study of their structural role in nerve membranes, qualitatively and quantitatively very important, has been neglected [1]. The dietary polyunsaturated fatty acids, linoleic and linolenic acid, are the necessary precursors of longer chains. The latter control the composition

---

[1] This work was supported by INSERM, INRA, CETIOM and ONIDOL.
[2] Abbreviations used:
    18:2 n–6: linoleic acid
    18:3 n–3: linolenic acid
    20:4 n–6: arachidonic acid
    22:6 n–3: cervonic acid, docosahexaenoic acid
    ERG: electroretinogram

of membranes, hence their fluidity, and in consequence the enzymatic activities, the binding between molecules and receptors, the cellular interactions, and the transport of nutrients.

The nervous system is the organ with the greatest concentration of lipids, immediately after adipose tissue. These lipids are practically all structural and not energetic, they participate directly in the functioning of cerebral membranes. Cerebral development is genetically programmed: if one stage is missed or perturbed, the chances of recuperation are greatly reduced. Moreover, the renewal of neurons and oligodendrocytes is practically nil (a cell that disappears is not replaced), the renewal of membranes is often very slow.

It is therefore necessary to ensure that these cells receive adequate supplies, especially of lipids, during their differentiation and multiplication. A lipidic anomaly could result in altered function of the membranes and a greater susceptibility of the membranes to aggression, particularly toxic.

It is well known that dietary polyunsaturated fatty acids control fatty acids in the membranes [2] and that they are particularly important for harmonious cerebral development [3].

The fatty acids participate in the structure of phospholipids but not that of sphingolipids. In the nervous system, on average, one fatty acid out of four is polyunsaturated. Results demonstrating the influence of polyunsaturated fatty acids on the structure and function of the nervous system are thus numerous [4-16]. However, these authors have generally used diets simultaneously deficient in fatty acids of the n–6 and n–3 series. Deficiency in all the essential fatty acids changes the course of cerebral development, period when nutrient requirements are particularly important. Nervous tissue compensates partially for this deficit by synthesizing polyunsaturated acids of the n–9 series which it incorporates in all its membranes.

The very long chain cerebral polyunsaturated fatty acids are derived from precursors that have a dietary origin. Polyunsaturated fatty acids of the n–3 series have a very specific role in the membranes, especially in the nervous system: all the cells and cerebral organelles are extremely rich in them. If animals are given diets containing variable quantities of linoleic and linolenic acids, there is (figure 1) a certain homeostasis of fatty acids of the n–6 series in serum, in contrast, serum levels of n–3 acids are in close correlation with dietary content. It is therefore extremely important to know precisely the amount of linolenic acid needed in the diet, because serum levels and consequently the composition of nervous membranes can depend on it.

Materials and methods

We used two groups of wistar rats. One group was fed for four generations with a semi synthetic diet containing 1.5% sunflower seed oil (1 000 mg of n–6 fatty acids and 6 mg of n–3 fatty acids). The other group was fed with soybean oil diet (1 000 mg n–6 fatty acids, and 135 mg per 100 g) or rapeseed oil (1 000 mg n–6 fatty

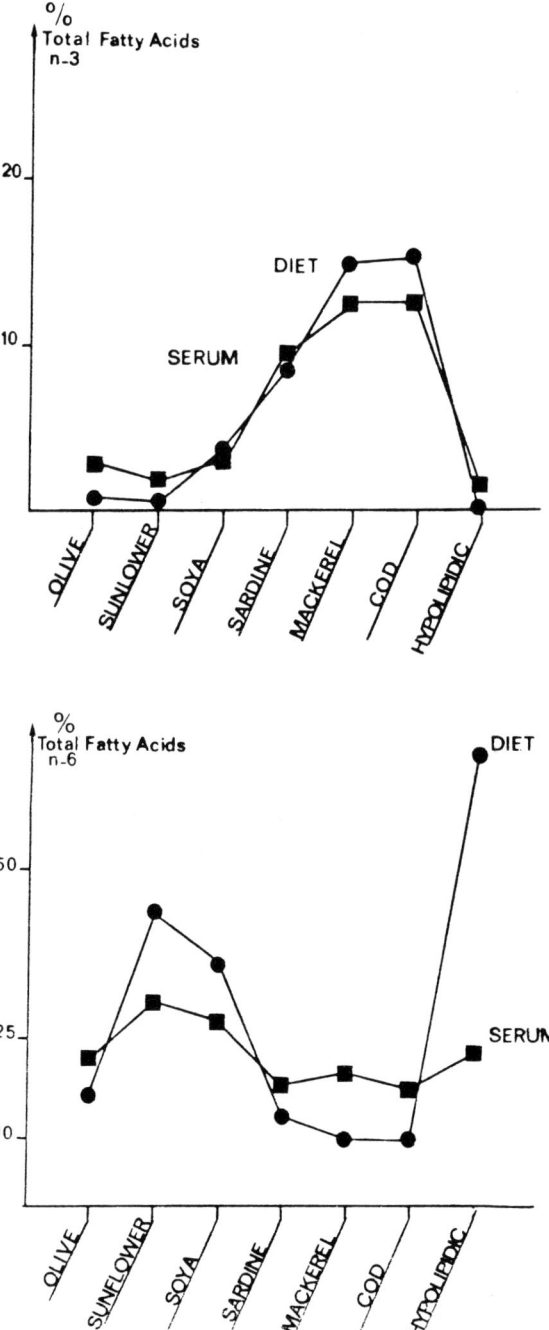

Figure 1. Correlation between dietary 18:2 and 18:3 and serum polyunsaturated fatty acids. (Data from Durand).

acids, and 250 mg n–3 fatty acids per 100 g). For animals given the "sunflower" diet, perinatal mortality has been found to be abnormally high [17]. three days after parturition, litters were adjusted to 10 animals. At 60 days after birth, animals receiving the "sunflower" diet were changed to a "soybean" or to a "rapeseed" diet in order to study the rate of recuperation as from the 60th day. Diets intermediate in linolenic acid content were obtained by adding variable and increasing amounts of linolenic acid by addition of rapeseed or soybean oil to the peanut or sunflower diet. Diet intermediate in linoleic acid content were obtained by adding variable amount of linseed oil, and palm oil to rapeseed oil or sunflower oil. Thus in these experiments linolenic acid content varied from 6 to 681 mg/100 g diet and linoleic acid from 150 to 6200 mg/100 g diet. Four weeks before mating these diets were given to females previously fed with sunflower oil. Their pups were sacrified when 21 days-old and 60 days-old.

Separation of neurons, oligodendrocytes, astrocytes, myelin, nerve endings (synaptic vesicles), mitochondria, endoplasmic reticulum (microsomes) has been previously described. The purity of fractions was evaluated by phase-contrast microscopy, enzyme marker assay, specific protein analysis (radioimmunoassay), electrophoresis, and lipid analysis [18]. Brain capillaries were prepared according to Goldstein [19] and their purity checked [20]. Extraction methods for lipid fractions, their transmethylation and the analysis of methyl esters by capillary column gas chromatography have also been previously described [18].

Electroretinogram recordings were performed as previously published [21].

The shuttle box text (measuring learning capacities) is a test of conditioning whose purpose is to measure learning capacity. A cage was divided into two compartments with a connecting hatch, one had an electrifiable floor and a roof lamp. Ten seconds after the roof lamp lit, electric current was applied in the compartment occupied. The test lasted 15 min and two shocks were delivered each minute. The conditioning of an animal was judged by the speed with which it passed from one compartment to the other after the lamp had lit in order to avoid the shock. Each test period therefore gave three different types of result: the number of non-passages (the animal having remained in the same compartment despite the electric current right up till the extinction of the light and termination of the electric shock); the number of passages with shock (the animal having reacted to the light signal but was unable to escape the shock for a more or less longer period of time); the number of passages without shock which was the number of avoidances (the animal having made the connection between the light and the shock and was thus able to avoid it).

Resistance to poisons (triethyltin): triethyltin was made up in physiologic solution and administered at a dosage of 0.5 ml/100 g body weight. The product was administered by the intraperitoneal route in one single dose to animals that had been fasted for 16 hours and had been under observation for 8 days. Determination of the LD 50 was made after establishment of the LD 0 and LD 100 and of intermediate doses chosen in geometric progression.

Results and discussion

Deficiency in linolenic acid produced anomalies in the composition of cells and organelles in the nervous system as well as in other organs

In animals fed the sunflower diet, cells and organelles show a very marked deficit in cervonic acid (22:6 n–3) that is compensated by an excess of 22:5 n–6. If 60 days old animals fed either the sunflower or soybean diet are compared, the total n –3/n–6 ratio is 16 times less in the oligodendrocytes, 12 times less in myelin, 2 times less in neurons, 6 times less in synaptic vesicles, 3 times less in astrocytes, 7 times less in mitochondria, and 5 times less in microsomes. Cells and intracellular organelles in all dietary group are found to have an identical total amount of polyunsaturated fatty acids with the two diets. Saturated and monounsaturated fatty acids are practically unchanged. Specific alterations in 22:6 n–3 and 22:5 n–6 are shown in *Table I*.

Table I. Amounts of 22:6 n–3 and 22:5 n–6 in "sunflower" animals expressed as % of "soybean" animals

	$\frac{\text{Sunflower}}{\text{Soybean}} \times 100$	
	18:3 n – 3	18:2 n – 6
Diet	4	101
	22:6 n – 3	22:5 n – 6
Neurons	48	214
Nerve endings	27	1 088
Oligodendrocytes	10	240
Myelin	14	1 200
Astrocytes	47	344
Mitonchondria	25	917
Microsomes	28	592
Retina	36	1 280
Capillaries	26	362
Sciatic nerve	28	1 000
Liver	40	560

Effect of "soybean" and "sunflower" diets on the 22:6 n – 3 and 22:5 n – 6 content of cells and cerebral organelles. Same remarks as in Fig. 2 and 3.

Even though the brain is considered to be the most protected organ in the body, faced with a deficiency in linolenic acid the membranes of cerebral cells and organelles are just as deficient, if not more so, as those of other organs. In any case, there is large preservation of dietary linolenic acid (and a reutilization of its very long chain derivatives) because a 25-fold decrease in the diet only results in, at the worst, a 10-fold decrease in the fractions we have examined (*Table I*). The importance of fatty acids of the n–3 series can similarly be well demonstrated by specifically studying certain phospholipids such as phosphatidylethanolamine in animals fed diets based on peanut or rapeseed oils [22, 23].

After changing from the "sunflower" to the "soybean diet", the rate of recuperation is remarkably slow: several months are necessary before the cerebral cells (*figure 2*) and organelles recover their normal levels of cervonic acid and lose the excess 22:5 n–6 [24] in contrast with other organs such as liver (*figure 2*). This recuperation in brain is slow regardless of the cell or organelle. One might have foreseen that recuperation would not be rapid in myelin, a membrane with a slow rate of renewal. But it is very unexpected to find that nerve endings also recuperate very slowly, although the renewal of molecules comprising their membranes is supposed to be rapid. It can be proposed that the regulation of recuperation is situated either at the level of the hepatic production of chain terminals (cervonic and arachidonic acid), or at the level of the enzymatic activities of desaturation and elongation that are known to be very low in the brain after birth [9, 25], or at the level of transport across the blood-brain barrier.

In the sciatic nerve, the rate of recuperation (after changing from a diet deficient in linolenic acid to a normal diet) is also very slow [27].

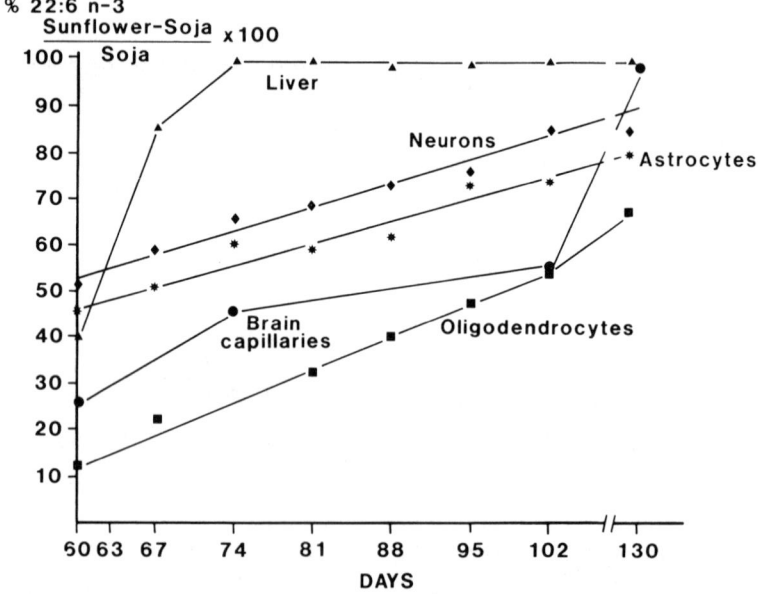

Figure 2. Rate of recuperation of cerebral organelles and cells in fatty acids. Comparison with other organs. The values were obtained by expressing the amounts of 22:6 n – 3 found in animals changed from sunflower to soybean diets at various times as a percentage of that found in animals fed the soybean diet continuously. This eliminates quantitative differences and permits easy comparison of recuperation rates. Deficient animals were fed a diet containing 940 mg/100 g diet 18:2 n–6 and 6 mg/100 g diet 18:3 n–3. For this recovery study they were fed a non deficient diet from 60 days (940 mg/100 g diet 18:2 n–6; 150 mg/100 g diet 18:3 n–3).

Cerebral microvessels and capillaries also have a very slow rate of recuperation (*figure 2*) even though they are in contact with in normal plasmatic lipoproteins.

Definition of the minimum necessary amount of n–3 fatty acids to assure normal composition of cerebral membranes

If diets that are intermediate in linolenic acid content (obtained by adding variable and increasing amounts of linolenic acid by addition of rapeseed or soybean oil to the peanut or sunflower diet) are given, increasing quantities of 18:3 n–3 results in an overall increase in all tissues studied of n–3 fatty acid very long chain (*figure 3*) and inversely a decrease in n–6 terminals (*figure 4*). In the whole brain organelles in myelin and nerve endings the level of 22:6 n–3 increases linearly for a 18:3 n – 3 intake varying from 0 to 200-250 mg/100 g of diet, it then reaches a plateau (the inverse is observed for 22:5 n–6). In the liver the response is rapid up to 300 mg per 100 g chow, beyond that point there is a slower increase. Very interestingly all organs examined need the same level of dietary linolenic acid (approx. 0.4% calories).

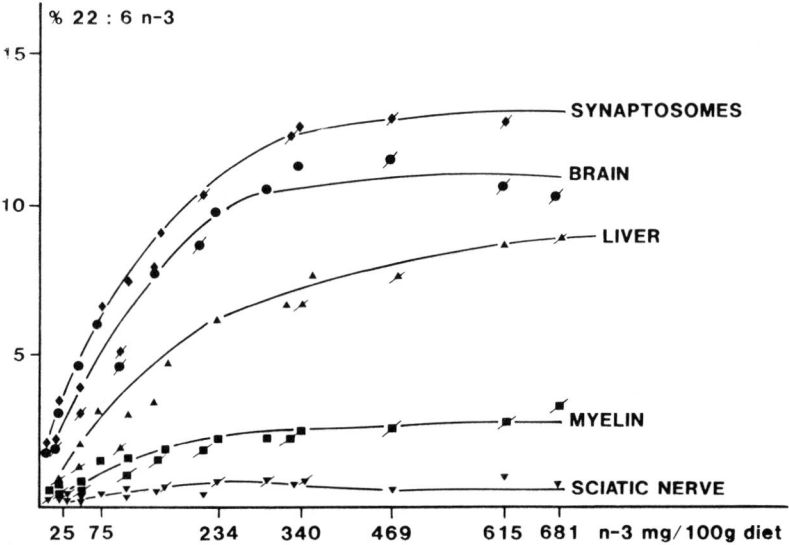

Figure 3. Relationship between dietary linolenic acid content and 22:6 n–3 levels in different organs and fractions. Animals were fed a diet containing 5 or 10% lipids (thus providing 2 levels of 18:2 n–6). 3 200 mg/100 g diet: normal symbols; 6 400 mg/100 g diet: symbols with a bar. Intermediate linolenic acid contents were obtained by adding increasing quantities of peanut oil to the rapeseed oil (or sunflower oil to soya oil). For brain liver, heart, kidney, muscle, adipose tissue, each point represent the mean value from at least 5 different preparations; each preparation needed at least 3 animals; thus each individual point was obtained from at least 15 animals. For myelin and synaptosome each point represent the mean value from at least 3 different preparations; each preparation needed at least 4 animals; thus each individual point was obtained from at least 12 animals. For sciatic nerve same remarks as in Fig. 2.

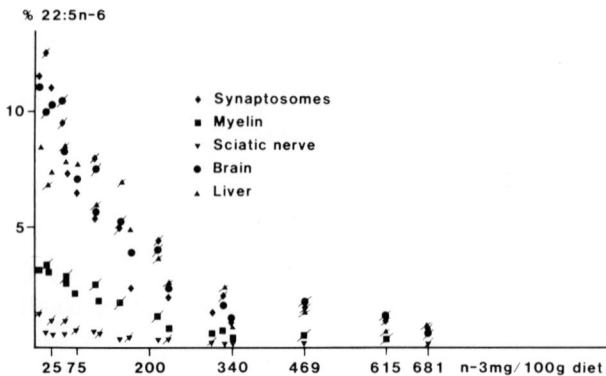

Figure 4. Relationship between dietary linolenic acid and 22:5 n–6 acid levels in different organs and fractions. Same remarks as in Fig. 3.

There is a direct relationship between dietary and gastric content in n–3 fatty acids. In serum, only the HDL (but not the LDL nor the VLDL) are enriched in n–3 with the diet. Study of the composition of lipoprotein polyunsaturated fatty acids demonstrates the importance of intrahepatic metabolism in the supply of polyunsaturated fatty acids to the brain; direct capture by the brain of 18:2 n–6 and 18:3 n–3 precursors is probably small. These precursors have to be desaturated and elongated in the liver to longer chains which are, in fact, the essential fatty acids for the brain [28], as appears to have been established by cell cultures [29]. The brain contains practically no linoleic or linolenic acid; cultured nerve cells can not synthesize measurable amounts of docosahexanoic acid (22:6 n–3). Only the addition of 20:4 n–6 and 22:6 n–3 to nerve cell culture medium results in, on the one hand, a better functioning of the neurons (measured, for example, by the renewed release of neurotransmitters) [30], and on the other, the multiplication and differentiation of oligodendrocytes thanks to a normal fatty acid composition of their membranes.

The linolenic acid requirements increase slightly with the dietary content of linoleic acid. For the developing brain in the rat, for 1 000, 2 500 and 5 000 mg/100 g 18:2 n–6, requirements in 18:3 n–3 are approximately 175, 200 and 250 mg/100 g respectively (*figure 4*).

Interestigly, increasing amount of 18:2 n–6 in the diet from 150 mg to 6 200 mg/100 g diet changed poorly the level of 22:6 n–3 in brain, sciatic nerve, myelin, nerve endings (*figure 5a*) as well as in various organs (*figure 5b*) except in adipose tissue. In fact increasing amount of 18:2 n–6 up to 300 – 1 400 mg/100 g diet (according to the organ) changed 20:4 n–6 content; after that it was a plateau, except in adipose tissue. Higher quantities of 18:2 n–6 in the diet only altered 22:5 n–6 and to a lesser extend 22:4 n–6. Thus the level of 22:6 n–3 and 20:4 n–6 are highly controlled by some unknown mechanism: defiency in n–3 fatty acids or excess of 18:2 n–6 both provoke accumulation of 22:5 n–6.

Excess dietary n–3 polyunsaturated fatty acids does not lead to an accumulation in the nervous system. In the brains of animals whose diet is enriched in n–3 fatty acid (5% lipid and 1% menhaden oil), the vitamin E, conjugated dienes, and malonaldehyde contents are not changed, nor are the glutathione peroxidase, catalase,

Minimum linolenic acid

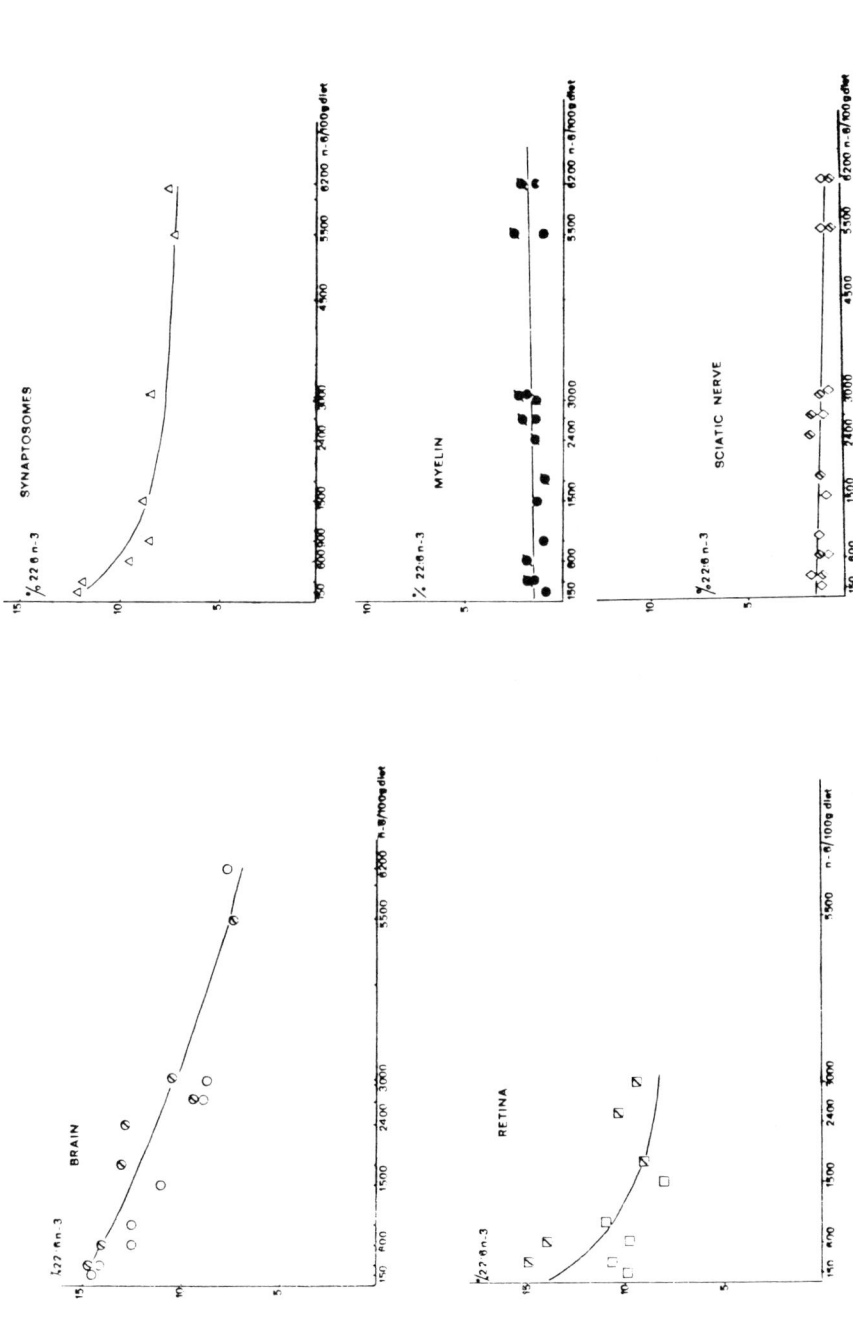

Figure 5. Relationship between dietary linoleic acid content and 22:6 n–3 level in organs. Animals were fed varying amount of 18:2 n–6 (from 150 mg to 6 200 mg/100 g diet); 18:3 n–3 was 150 mg for half the points (normal symbols), and 300 mg for the other half (symbols with a bar). Same remark as in Fig. 2 and 3 for number of animals of each point. Note that the scale for 18:2 n–6 is very large, in comparison the one for 22:6 n–3 is very small. Thus few percent alterations in membrane 22:6 n–3 are obtained when dietary 18:2 n–6 is increased by approx; 4 100%.

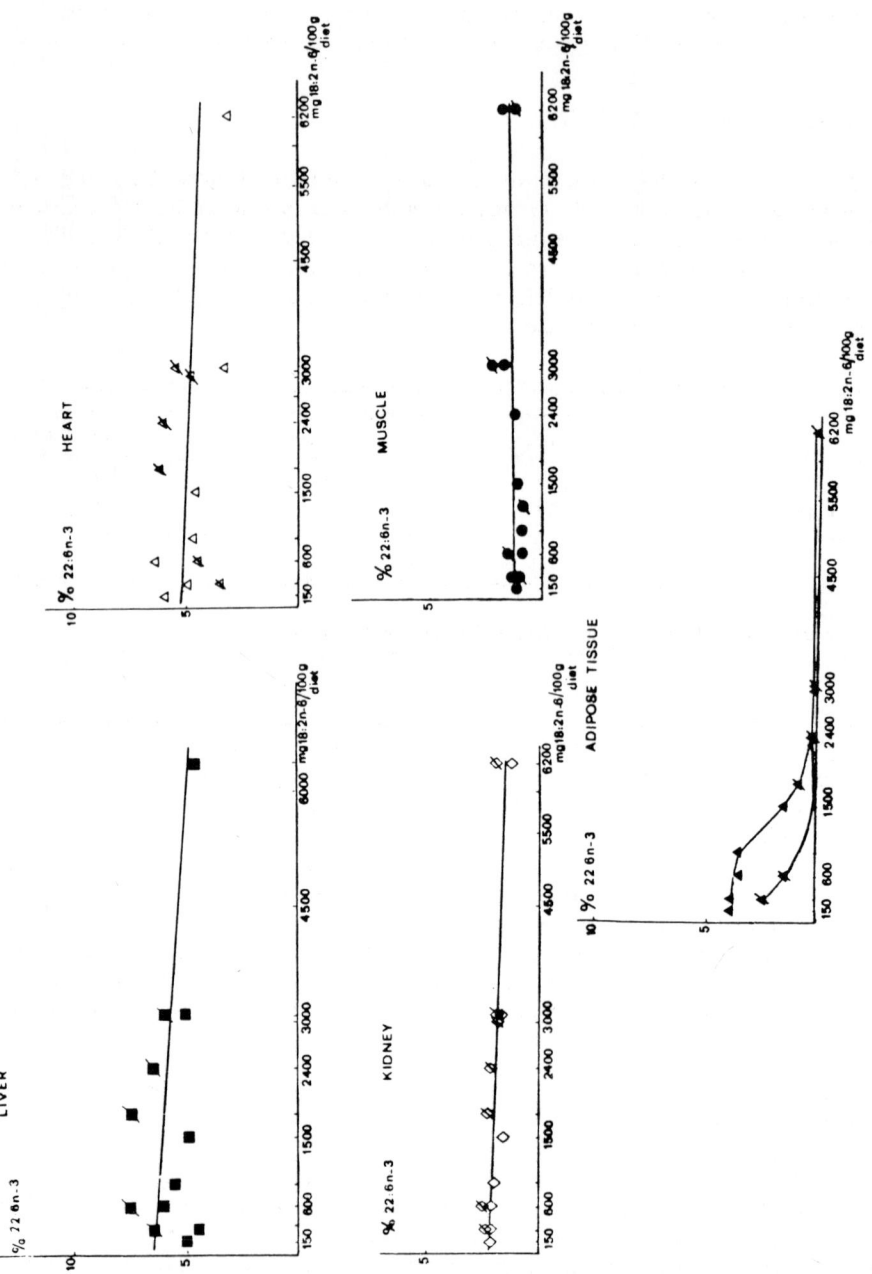

Figure 5b

and superoxide dismutase activities [31]. Slight excess fats are unlikely to be implicated in attacks by free radicals or to be broken down into toxic derivatives by peroxidation in the brain. However, feeding animal with large excess of fish oil (15% cod liver) alters C22:6 and C20:5 n–3 brain contents (unpublished data).

Enzymatic activities *(Table II)*

The activity of 5'-nucleotidase is decreased by 30% in total brain, but not in myelin nor in nerve terminals, which suggests that the enzyme in cellular membranes is probably very altered. These results are in agreement with those of Bernsohn *et al.* [32] who showed that the decrease in the activity of the enzyme produced by a simultaneous deficiency of linoleic and linolenic acids is corrected only by the addition of linolenic acid to the diet.

Table II. Decrease in membrane enzyme activities produced by a deficiency in linolenic acid

	Brain	Myelin	Nerve endings
5'-nucleotidase	0.70	0.94	1.20
Na$^+$K$^+$ATPase	0.95	1.10	0.55

Figures show the ratio of enzyme activities in "sunflower" animals to that in "soybean" animals.
Each value is the mean from is the mean from 4 preparations. Each preparation for myelin and nerve endings needed 10 animals.
Measurement of enzymatic activities was performed as previously described [54].

Na-K-ATPase is decreased by half in the nerve endings of animals fed a "sunflower" diet as compared to those fed a "soybean" diet, who show normal levels of enzyme activity. interestingly, a specific deficiency in linolenic acid produces a decrease in this enzymatic activity, while a simultaneous deficiency in linoleic and linolenic acids results in an increase in this same activity [16]. This enzyme, Na-K-ATPase, controls the ionic flow resulting from nerve transmission. It consumes half the energy used by the brain (in an adult man this organ only represents 2% of body weight but consumes 20% of energy).

Another enzyme, acetylcholinesterase, also has its activity modulated by dietary lipids [33]. The effects of the nature of membrane fatty acids on enzymatic activities have been studied in numerous organs [6, 34], thus the brain does not escape the general rule.

Electroretinogram

Substantial perturbations in the ERG of animals deficient in alpha-linolenic acid aged 4 weeks as seen in *figure 6*. In 4-week-old sunflower animals the *a* and *b* waves are only detectable at stimulation intensities that are ten times those of soybean fed animals. these perturbations begin to decline at the age of 6 weeks and disappear in adult (16 to 18 weeks), except for the *a* wave whose amplitude, at

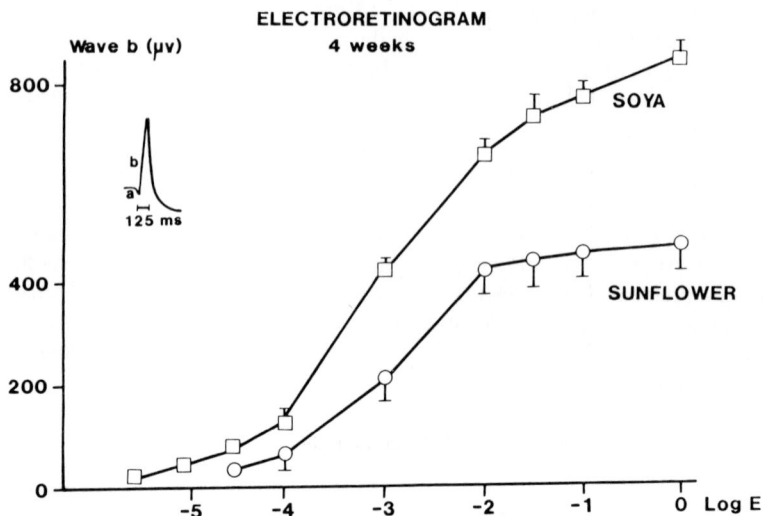

Figure 6. Electroretinogram *a* and *b* waves are altered in young animals deficient in linolenic acid. Each point is the mean value from at least 12 animals.

maximum stimulation intensity only, has a value 10% lower than that found in the control group, perhaps indicating an irreversible change.

Similarly in young animals (21 days) fed a "peanut" diet, the amplitude of the ERG is three times less than that obtained with animals fed a "rapeseed" diet [28].

The retina is one of the tissues that is richest in n–3 polyunsaturated fatty acids [5]. Overall deficiencies in polyunsaturated fatty acids induce, in the long term, modifications in the distribution of membrane fatty acids in the retina [35] which is related to perturbations in the amplitude of the *a* and *b* waves in the lectroretinogram [36]. But the direct influence of dietary fatty acids on the electroretinogram has been argued according to species, age, and the duation of the deficiency, and it has even been denied [37].

Learning text results

It is known that a deficiency in linoleic and linolenic acids alters the learning capacity of animals [15, 38, 39].

The learning behaviour of sunflower animals are very perturbed, as shown by the shuttle box test (*figure 7*). At the first test period it is clear that "soybean" animals made a quicker association between the light signal and the electric shock, since on average they avoid 7 shocks out of 30, while the "sunflower" animals only avoided 2. The number of passages with shock is the same in both groups, but the number of non-passages is much higher in the "sunflower" group. This means that "sunflower" animals undergo electric shock for the whole duration of the stimulus without attempting, or without being able, to escape. The "soybean" animals total

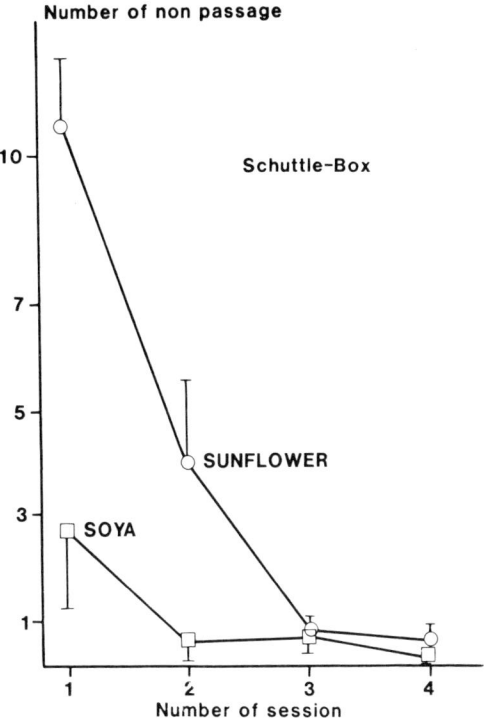

Figure 7. Perturbation of learning tests (shuttle box) in animals deficient in linolenic acid. Each point is the mean value from at least 15 animals.

2 non-passages out of 30 stimulations while "sunflower" animals total 10. As a function of the number of test periods differences tend to decline and disappear at the fourth test period. Learning impairment in "sunflower" animals could be related to a decrease in learning capacity, but also to more intense emotivity. These results are in agreement with those of Lamptey and Walker [40].

Less rapid mortality in animals not deficient in linolenic acid when tested with a neurotoxic agent, triethyltin

The animals given the "sunflower" diet die more rapidly than those given the "soybean" diet (*figure 8*). Although the LD 50 of animals given the "soybean" or "sunflower" diets does not differ significantly (6.18 versus 6.02 µl/kg). The nature of the polyunsaturated fatty acids can therefore, affect the process of detoxification at the level of hepatic membranes [41] and also make the cerebral membranes more fragile.

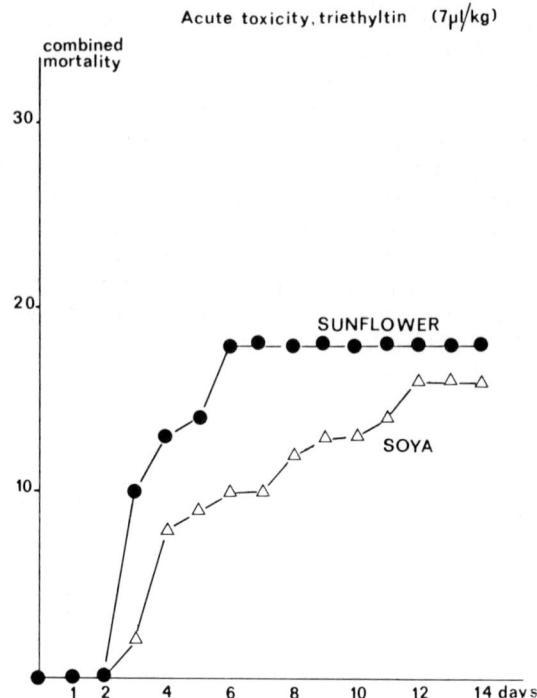

Figure 8. A neurotoxic agent (acute triethyltin) is more rapidly fatal in "sunflower" animals than in "soybean" animals.

Conclusions

A pathogenesis of linolenic acid deficiency has been described in the monkey [42], and in man [14, 43, 44]. A syndrome of modern society has been proposed as being a deficiency in series n–3 fatty acids [45]. It is, therefore, certainly very important to verify exactly the amout of n–3 acids in the diet: a minimum must be supplied to allow cerebral membranes to have a normal composition and function: 200 mg/100 g food intake is a minimum in the developing animal, hence also in man. Thus, this work recommend that alpha-linolenic acid represent 0.4% of the total dietary calories, in agreement with studies in animal [46] as well as in human [14, 47, 48].

Requirements in n–3 acids are very high in man during the neonatal period [7, 8] and must be supplied to the mother during gestation, then to the newborn. It should be remarked that human milk contains non-negligible amounts of linolenic acid, and also of cervonic acid, which are sometimes absent from artificial milks. Human newborns receiving artificial milk have red blood cells that are deficient in cervonic acid [49] and the fatty acid composition of red blood cells can serve as an index of cerebral membrane composition [50]. In addition, there is incontestably a relationship between dietary lipids and the properties of red blood cells [51].

The origin of brain saturated and unsaturated fatty acid (in situ synthesis and nutritional origin) is well documented [52]; in contrast polyunsaturated fatty acid metabolism in nervous tissue needs further studies.

Polyunsaturated fatty acid deficiencies can appear among the newborn fed with artificial milk, the inhabitants of the Third World (in children but also in adults), in the elderly on special diets, in invalids (enteral and parenteral nutrition), and in surgical patients whose requirements are often increased. This study shows that dietary linolenic requirement to synthesize membranes is the same whatever the organ (200 mg/100 g diet). In contrast linoleic requirement vary between 150 and 1 200 mg/100 diet food according to the organ (data to be published). Thus the optimum dietary n–6/n–3 ratio is between 1 and 6 according to the organ. Thus we suggest that minimum linolenic and linoleic acid in the diet to be 200 mg and 1 200 mg/100 g diet, i.e. 0.4% and 2.4% calories.

Acknowledgements

This work was supported by INSERM, INRA, CETIOM, ONIDOL. The authors are greatful to Michelle Bonneil for typing this manuscript.

References

1. Mead J.F. (1984) The non-eicosanoid functions of the essential fatty acids. *J. Lipid Res.* 25: 1517-1521.
2. Holman R.T. (1986) Control of polyunsaturated acids in tissue lipids. *J. Amer. Col. Nutr.* 5: 183-211.
3. Menon N.K., Dhopeshwarkar G.A. (1982) Essential fatty acid deficiency and brain development. *Prog. Lipid Res.* 21: 309-326.
4. Alling C., Bruce A., Karlsson I., Sapia O., Svennerholm L.J. (1971) Effect of maternal essential fatty acid supply on fatty acid composition of brain, liver, muscle and serum in 21-day-old rats. *J. Nutr.* 102: 773-782.
5. Bazan N., Di Fazio De Escalante S., Careaga M., Bazan H.E.P, Giusto N.M. (1982) High content of 22:6 (docosahexaenoate) and active (2-^{3}H) glycerol metabolism of phosphatidic acid from photoreceptor membranes. *Biochim. Biophys. Acta* 712: 702-706.
6. Brenner R.R. (1984) Effect of unsaturated acids on membrane structure and enzyme kinetics. *Prog. Lipid Res.* 23: 69-96.
7. Clandinin M.T., Chappell J.E., Leong S., Heim T., Swyer P.R., Chance G.W. (1980) Intrauterine fatty acid accretion rates in human brain: implications for fatty acid requirements. *Early Human Development,* 4/2: 121-129.
8. Clandinin M.T., Chappell J.E., Leong S., Heim T., Swyer P.R., Chance G.W. (1980) Extrauterine fatty acid accretion in infant brain: implication for fatty acid requirements. *Early Human Development* 4/2: 131-138.
9. Cook H.W. (1978) *In vitro* formation of polyunsaturated fatty acids by desaturation in rat brain: some properties of the enzyme in developing brain and comparison with liver. *J. Neurochem.* 30: 1327-1334.
10. Crawford M.A., Sinclair A.J. (1971) *Nutritional influences in the evolution of mammalian brain.* A Ciba Foundation Symposium, ASP, Elsevier. Excerpta Medical, North-Holland, Amsterdam. pp. 267-292.

11. Crawford M.A., Hassam A.G., Stevens P.A. (1981) Essential fatty acid requirements in pregnancy and lactation with special reference to brain development. *Prog. Lipid Res.* 20: 31-40.
12. Dhopeshwarkar G.A., Mead J.F. (1973) Uptake and transport of fatty acids into the brain and the role of the blood-brain barrier system. *Adv. Lipid Res.* 11: 109-142.
13. Holman R.T. (1968) Essential fatty acid deficiency. In: *Progress in the Chemistry of Fats and Other Lipids*. 9, Part. 2. pp. 279. R.T. Holman (ed). Pergamon Press, Oxford (England).
14. Holman R.T., Johnson S.B., Hatch T.F. (1982) A case of human linolenic acid deficiency involving neurological abnormalities. *Am. J. Clin. Nutr.* 35: 617-623.
15. Paoletti R., Galli C. (1972) Effect of essential fatty acid deficiency on the central nervous system in the growing rat. In: *Lipid Malnutrition and the Developing Brain*. Ciba Foundation Symposium, pp. 121-140.
16. Sun G.Y., Sun A.Y. (1974) Synaptosomal plasma membranes: acyl group composition of phosphoglycerides and ($Na^+ + K^+$)-ATPase activity during fatty acid deficiency. *J. Neurochem.* 22: 15-18.
17. Guenest Ph., Pascal G., Durand G. (1986) Dietary alpha-linolenic acid deficiency in the rat effects on reproduction and post natal growth. *Reprod. Nutr. Develop.* 28: 969-985.
18. Bourre J.M., Pascal G., Durand G., Masson M., Dumont O., Piciotti, M. (1984) Alterations in the fatty acid composition of rat brain cells (neurons, astrocytes and oligodendrocytes) and of subcellular fractions (myelin and synaptosomes) induced by a diet devoid of n–3 fatty acids. *J. Neurochem.* 43: 342-348.
19. Goldstein G.W. (1979) Relation of potassium transport to oxidative metabolism in isolated brain capillaries. *J. Physiol.* 286: 185-195.
20 Homayoun P., Roux F., Niel E., Bourre J.M. (1985) The synthesis of lipids from ($1 - ^{14}C$) acetate by isolated rat brain capillaries. *Neurosci. Lett.* 62: 143-147.
21. Weidner C. (1981) The presence of an albino ERG in the pigmented rat: genetic implications. *J. Physiol.* 77: 813-821.
22. Nouvelot A., Bourre J.M., Sezille G., G., Dewailly P., Jaillard J. (1983) Changes in the fatty acid patterns of brain phospholipids during development of rats fed peanut or rapeseed oil, taking into account differences between milk and maternal food. *Ann. Nutr. Metabol.* 27: 233-241.
23. Nouvelot A., Delbart C., Bourre J.M. (1986) Hepatic metabolism of dietary alpha-linolenic acid in suckling rats, and its possible importance in polyunsaturated fatty acid uptake by the brain. *Ann. Nutr. Metab.* 30: 316-323.
24. Youyou A., Durand G., Pascal G., Piciotti M., Dumont O., Bourre J.M. (1986) Recovery of altered fatty acid composition induced by a diet devoid or n–3 fatty acids in myelin, synaptosomes, mitochondria and microsomes of developing rat brain. *J. Neurochem.*, 46: 224-228.
25. Strouve-Vallet, Pascaud M. (1971) Désaturation de l'acide linoléique par les microsomes du foie et du cerveau du rat en développement. *Biochimie* 53: 699-703.
26. Homayoun P., Durand G., Pascal G., Bourre J.M. Alteration in fatty acid composition of adult rat brain capillaries and choroid plexus induced by a diet deficient in (– 3) fatty acids. Slow recovery by substitution with a non deficient diet. *J. Neurochem.* (in press).
27. Bourre J.M., Youyou A., Durand G., Pascal G. (1987) Slow recovery of the fatty acid composition of sciatic nerve in rats fed a diet initially low in n–3 fatty acids. *Lipids* 22: 535-537.
28. Nouvelot A., Dedonder E., Dewailly Ph., Bourre J.M. (1985) Influence des n–3 exogènes sur la composition en acides gras polyinsaturés de la rétine. Aspects structural et physiologique. *Cah. Nutr. Diét.* XX, 2: 123-125.
29. Bourre J.M., Faivre A., Dumont O. *et al.*, (1983) Effect of polyunsaturated fatty acids on fetal mouse brain cells in culture in a chemically defined medium. *J. Neurochem.* 41, 1234-1242.

30. Loudes C., Faivre A., Barret A., Grouselle D., Puymirat J. Tixier-Vidal M. (1983) Release of immunoreactive TRH in serum free culture of mouse hypothalamic cells. *Dev. Brain Res.* 9: 231-234.
31. Chaudière J., Clément M., Driss F., Bourre J.M. (1987) Unaltered brain membranes after prolonged intake of highly oxidizable long-chain fatty acids of the (n–3) series. *Neurosci. Lett.* (in press).
32. Bernshohn J., Spitz F.J. (1974) Linoleic and linolenic acid dependency of some brain membrane-bound enzymes after lipid deprivation in rats. *Biochem. Biophys. Res. Com.* 57: 293-298.
33. Foot M., Cruz T.F., Clandinin M.T. (1982) Influence of dietary fat on the lipid composition of rat brain synaptosomal and microsomal membranes. *Biochem. J.* 208: 631-640.
34. Farias R.N. (1980) Membrane cooperative enzymes as a tool for the investigation of membrane structure and related phenomena. *Lipid Res.* 17: 251-282.
35. Tinoco J., Miljanich P., Medwadowski B. (1977) Depletion of docosahexaenoic acid in retinal lipids of rats fed a linolenic acid-deficient, linoleic acid-containing diet. *Biochim. Biophys. Acta* 486: 575-578.
36. Neuringer M., Connor W.E. (1986) n-3 fatty acids int he brain and retina: evidence for their essentiality. *Nutr. Rev.* 44: 289.
37. Leat W.M.F., Curtis R., Millichamp N.J., Cox R.W. (1986) Retinal function in rats and guinea-pigs. Reared on diets low in essential fatty acids and supplemented with linoleic or linolenic acids. *Ann. Nutr. Metab.* 30: 166-174.
38. Caldwell mJ.A., Churchill J.A. (1966) Learning impairment in rats administered a lipid free diet during pregnancy. *Psychol. Rep.* 19: 99-102.
39. Lamptey M.S., Walker B.L. (1978) Learning behaviour and brain lipid composition in rats subjected to essential fatty acid deficiency during gestation. Lactation and growth. *J. Nutr.* 108: 358-367.
40. Lamptey M., Walker B.K. (1976) A possible essential role for dietary linolenic acid in the development of the young rat. *J. Nutrition* 106: 86-93.
41. Hammer C., Wills E.D. (1979) The effect of dietary fats on the composition of the liver endoplasmic reticulum and oxidative drug metabolism. *Br. J. Nutr.* 41: 465.
42. Fiennes R.N.T., Sinclair A.J., Crawford M.A. (1973) Essential fatty acid studies n primates linolenic acid requirements of capuchins. *J. Med. Prim.* 2: 155-169.
43. Anonymous (1986) Combined EFA deficiency in a patient on long term TPN. *Nutr. Rev.* 44: 301-305.
44. Bjerne K.S., Mostad I.L., Thoresen L. (1987) Alpha-linolenic acid deficiency in patients on long term gastric tube feeding: estimation of linolenic acid and long-chain unsaturated n–3 fatty acid requirement in man. *Scand. Am. J. Clin. Nutr.* (in press).
45. Rudin D. (1982) the dominant diseases of modernized societies as omega-3 essential fatty acid deficiency syndrome: substrate beriberi. *Med. Hypotheses.* 8: 17-47.
46. Pudelkewicz C., Seufert J., Holman R.T. (1968) Requirements of the female rat for linoleic and linolenic acids. *J. Nutr.* 94: 138-146 (1988).
47. Lasserre M., Mendy F., Spielmann D., Jacotot B. (1985) Effects of different dietary intake of essential fatty acids on C20:3 w6 and C20:4 w6 serum levels in human adult. *Lipids* 4: 227-233.
48. Kinsella J.E. (1986) Food components with potential therapeutic benefits: the n–3 polynsaturated fatty acids of fish oils. *Food Technology* 89-97.
49. Putnam J.C., Carlson S.E., De Voe P.W., Barness L.A. (1982) The effect of variations in dietary fatty acids on the fatty acid composition of erythrocyte phosphatidylcholine and phosphatidylethanolamine in human infants. *Amer. J. Clin. Nutr.* 36: 106-114.
50. Carlson S.E., Carver J.D., House S.G. (1986) high fat diets varying in ratios of polyunsaturated to saturated fatty acid and linoleic to linolenic acid: a comparison of rat neural and red cell membrane phospholipids. *J. Nutr.* 116: 718-725.

51. Popp-Snijders C., Schouten J.AZ., De Jong A.P., Van Der Veen, E.A. (1984) Effect of dietary cod-liver oil on thelipid composition of human erythrocyte membranes. *Scand. J. Clin. Lab. Invest.* 44: 39-46.
52. Bourre, J.M. (1980) Origin of aliphatic chains in brain. In: *Neurological Mutations Affecting Myelination.* N. Baumann (ed.) INSERM Symposium n° 14. Elsevier/North Holland Biomedical Press pp. 187-206.
53. Bourre J.M., Durand G., Pascal G., Youyou A. (1987) Recovery of altered polyunsaturated fatty acid composition induced by a diet deficient in n–3 fatty acids in brain cells (neurons, astrocytes and oligodendrocytes). Comparison with other organs. *J. Nutr.* (submitted).
54. Bourre J.M., Chanez C., Dumont O., Flexor, M.A. (1982) Alteration of 5'-nucleotidase and Na^+, K^+ ATPase in central and peripheral nervous tissue from dysmyelinating mutants (Jimpy, Quaking, Trembler, Shiverer and mld). Comparison with CNPase in the developing sciatic nerve from Trembler. *J. Neurochem.* 38: 643-649.

Summary

Feeding animals with oils that have a low linolenic acid content results in serious anomalies in the brain. In all brain cells and organelles reduced amount of 22:6 n – 3 is compensated by increase in 22:5 n – 6. Similar results are found in the liver. The speed at which it recuperates from these anomalies is extremely slow for brain cells, organelles and microvessels, in contrast with the liver. The nervous system is not heavily protected against deficiency nor has it priority in the satisfaction of its needs. Essential fatty acids for the brain could be those with very long chains as shown in cell culture. They are probably synthetized in the liver from linolenic acid. They can also be supplied directly by food. During the period of cerebral development there is a linear relation between the n – 3 acid content of the brain and that of food until linolenic acid represents approx. 200 mg per 100 g of food (for 1 100 mg linoleic acid). Beyond that point there is a plateau in the brain. Thus dietary requirements during brain development represent 0.4% calories for 18:3 n – 3 and 2.2% calories for 18:2 n – 6. These values are also correct for the liver. The level of 22:6 n – 3 in membranes is poorly affected by the dietary quantity of 18:2 n – 6 if at least 18:3 n – 3 represent 0.4% calories. A decrease in acids of the linolenic series in the membranes results in a 40% reduction of Na-K-ATPase in nerve terminals and a 20% reduction in 5'-nucleotidase in whole brain homogenate. A diet low in linolenic acid leads to anomalies in the electroretinogram which disappear partially with age has little effect on motor activity but it seriously affects learning tasks (altering emotivity). The presence of linolenic acid in the diet confers a greater resistance to certain neurotoxic agents (triethyltin, for example).

In view of the relative metabolism of man and the experimental model animal, their rates of development, their brain body ratios, and the fatty acid composition of their nerve membranes it is possible to suppose that results obtained in the rat are also valid for human.

Discussion

Dr Martinez: I agree very much with your point on the essentiality of linolenic acid, I wanted to know if you had used only linolenic acid, I mean only vegetable oils for your experiments with rats?

Dr Bourre: You mean if we have done experiments with only linolenic acid in the diet?

Dr Martinez: Yes, just only the parents I mean, no if you have used only the vegetable oils and not the long PUFA?

Dr Bourre: We are currently doing those kind of experiments and I would like to make some collaboration with some industry for that; because this is very important, because you provide DHA and EPA in the same time and in terms of nutrition EPA does devoid lipogenesis and DHA is very important to be incorporated into the cell membranes, which means that it's probably not excellent to give in the same time those two fatty acids, at least in terms of membrane function. And the other point is providing long chains, then you come back to a very old story which is the yellow fat disease which is a disease with oxidation of these very long chain which was obtained in animals and it's very well known and it is partly due to an excess of linolenic, an excess of EPA and DHA and a reduced amount of tocopherol for instance.

Dr Martinez: Probably the rat has a better system, delta 6 desaturase system, that's the difference I think with humans.

IDr Bourre: So it means once more if working with the rat it will be the same with human, which needs eventually more linolenic acid in comparison with rat.

Chairman: That's a very important point because enzymatic equipment of the rat is totally different from humans and so the point you made I think it's very relevant and perhaps you should just comment this a little bit more. Has any one questions?

Dr Cunnane: It's indirectly related, I think the evidence we have right now suggests that in adults there is negligeable desaturase activity at least it's been extremely difficult to prove it with supplementation studies, stable isotope studies, but we don't know what's happening at the stage of brain development in the first five years of life, whether the infant in fact has got substantial desaturase activity, that really remains an open question as far as I'm aware.

Dr Bourre: At least in the brain it has been published by three persons that the desaturase does dramatically goes down in rat for instance within few days during around birth. So few days after birth the activity is just negligeable to a certain extent.

Essential fatty acids

Dr Bjerve: I would comment on your comment on the yellow fatty disease and on the role of the lack of tocopherol or the increased need of tocopherol when you supply these fatty acids. I think we are talking about extremely small amounts of these fatty acids. The yellow fat disease, you only see it if you have bad fat preparations or and if you give them in large quantities. So I think we shall not be too cautious about these extremely small amounts of very long chain fatty acids which we probably are talking about if we're going to include, what we really are discussing is do we need to include some of the very long chain fatty acids of the type arachidonic acid or the type eicosapentanoic acid, docosahexanoic acid in the diets for specific types of diseases, human diseases and we don't know that at present, we have to find it out and I don't think we shall be too frightened about this increased need of tocopherol I don't think so, thank you.

Dr Bourre: You don't think we have not to be frightened about the amount of tocopherol?

Dr Bjerve: I don't think that's a practical problem.

Dr Bourre: This is a very important problem.

Dr Adam: We need to supply the tocopherol of course but it's possible to do it, and I think it is possible to make the preparations containing very small amounts also of the long chain fatty acids, if we need to.

Dr Bourre: So I would say that in fact you have to consider both linolenic acid and DHA. The organism does control the chain length so if overfeeding the animal with DHA or EPA then you bypass this control and then you can get some toxicology. Part of the toxicology is due to the reduced amount of tocopherol, reduced amount of protection against peroxidation but the situation is not clear because in fact it is not known exactly, it is not known at all in the membrane how polyunsaturated fatty acids are protected against peroxidation. You have one tocopherol per many hundred polyunsaturated fatty acids, and one thing the tocopherol does protect linolenic acid and arachidonic acid, it has been published by many authors. What about the protection for the linolenic series which is very important in any membrane, so it's not clear.

Chairman: So it's a very important question, the question was, is it necessary to include into the enteral or parenteral nutrition long chain fatty acids, that means arachidonic acid or eicosapentanoic acid and I think that's an open question.

Dr Bjerve: Just to say a few words, I agree with you that one should be cautious when preparing those kinds of formulas but we must not get into the same type of picture as we did when omega 6 were established as essential. Because you could not cure omega 6 fatty acid essential deficiency symptoms as efficient by supplying omega 3s; omega 3s were considered non-essential for decades in man. I think we shall not now stop this search or exploitation about what kind of fatty acids do we really need to supply to the critical ill man, be it preterm infants or extremely old and sick people. I think we shall not only talk about linoleic/linolenic we should also try to find, do we really need to also supply small amounts? Of let's say arachidonic? Let's say eicosapentanoic? I don't know, no one knows at present but I think it's important for those people having those illnesses that we finally find that out.

Chairman: So in summary one could say that linoleic acid and alphalinolenic acid serves function as EFAs, whereas the function of arachidonic acid and eicosapentanoic acid may be pharmaceutical; that means the functions in certain states like critical ill patients or rhumatism and so on, maybe it's this way?

Dr Bourre: Yes but you just have to add that DHA, which is just after EPA acid very important structural role for the moment in a membrane maybe some other roles which are unknown.

Prof Ghisolfi: What do you think about the time necessary to observe significant-linoleic acid deficiency state in infants. Have you any idea?

Dr Bourre: I'm not a clinician, so I ask you the question?

Prof Ghisolfi: No, but compared to rats.

Dr Bourre: I don't know. Just coming back to the skin symptoms we have to remind the communication by Dr Hansen. In fact in the skin you only have linoleic acid in these acylglucosylceramides so linolenic acid has just no role, in the skin, so why looking for linolenic on the skin because there it has no role? So it's not the response, it's another point in fact.

Dr Hansen: I think that linoleic acid is essential, arachidonic acid is essential, they have each their functions. DHA is probably also essential for functioning, probably also EPA, but is alphalinolenic acid essential in its own right or is it just precursor, have you any comment on that?

Dr Bourre: Well, I don't know, for the moment I would say both.

Dr Hansen: Why?

Dr Bourre: Because we have no experiments with DHA and it's very difficult.

Dr Hansen: Yes, but you find EPA in the tissue but you do not find alphalinolenic acid.

Dr Bourre; For the moment I would say both because we have just results with alphalinolenic and dietary experiments and cell culture with DHA, but this is not a right conclusion because you have the blood brain barrier, you have the synthesis by the liver during development, during ageing and the situation, you know it's obscure for the moment, So nobody knows; in fact, if the desaturase is reduced at a level which provides an enzymatic activity which is not sufficient to provide DHA, nobody knows, including during ageing, because this is very important for aged people to provide DHA just for the turnover of their membranes, any membranes including the brain.

Dr Cunnane: I think the issue that has just been raised, if we can spend a few minutes it would be worth while, because if you look at evolution for instance before there qas TPN, take our evolution over many, many thousands of years say even millions of years we could have had access to 22.6 and EPA to some extent. But we also had alpalinolenic acid from a very very long time and I think that this somehow is incorporated into our biological biochemical development such that our system will be able to tolerate a certain amount of 22.6, but it will equally prefer perhaps to deal with maybe 50% of omega 3s as alphalinolenic acid and synthesize the 22.6, because I think 33.6 could be toxic as well and we shouldn't be trying to rely on it being available as itself preformed as opposed to the synthetic route which the body has developed over many thousands of years to incorporate. So yes we can take fish oils but I don't think we can avoid the essentiality of alphalinolenic acid as precursor.

Chairman: One final question.

Dr Messing: It's not really a question but I am not a specialist in this field and after the past ten minutes, I'm completely lost now in omega 3 and omega 6 and so my question is: what is specific to omega 3 and what is specific to omega 6 in the brain membrane. In your opinion of course. What is specific about function concerning omega 3 or omega 6 in brain function?

Dr Bourre: So this could be the next step, for the moment the demonstration is that linolenic acid is used for the membrane and if today it is deficient then you have alterations in enzymatic activities, electrophysiology and learning performances, susceptibilities to neurotoxines. So the next step is what about the specificity and you have at least one aspect the 5 prime nucleotidase in the membrane is controlled only by linolenic acid, but this is not the right question as you can see, the right answer I would say.

Dr Messing: Yes it's only a part of the question because in your recommendation you do not talk only about omega 3 but also about omega 6, so what is specific concerning omega 6?

Dr Bourre: I don't know. If I understand the question which specific function in the brain is totally controlled by omega 3 fatty acids, I don't know, not yet.

Chairman: Perhaps Stephen Cunnane has given the answer already as a development of life coming from the sea and all those organs living in the sea depended on omega 3 fatty acids and then coming to the land got acquainted to omega 6 fatty acids and those ancient tissues originating from it.

4

Fatty acid composition of rat tissues during total parenteral nutrition (TPN)

F.M. MARTINS

Department of Paedriatric Surgery 54, Hospital D. Estefania, Lisboa, Portugal

Dr Martins: Mr Chairman, ladies and gentlemen, first of all I want to thank the organising committee and Prof Ghisolfi for the kind invitation to participate in this meeting. I'm supposed to speak about the fatty acid composition of different tissues in rats during total parenteral nutrition.

It is nowadays possible to feed intravenously most of the patients and it is a routine, it became a routine in almost all hospitals in the world. The risks are predictable and controllable, so why the rats? Well, for those of us who work with children the physiological response and the metabolic adaptation of the growing tissues to the administration of all the nutrients through the parenteral route remains still a question of debate.

Since experimental parenteral nutrition is not possible for ethical reasons in healthy children the animal model is, of course, the solution. Accordingly an experimental model was designed by us in collaboration with the Faculty of Medicine of Upsala and the Kabivitrum laboratories in Stockholm. The aim of the study was to investigate the effect of energy and energy substrate ration on growth and lipid composition of different fat tissues. We have studied four different fat to carbohydrate ratios and no fat group, and this is with regard to non-protein energy in which all the energy was given as glucose. A low fat group with supply of 6% of non-protein energy as fat, a medium fat group with 30% as fat and a high fat group with 60% as fat. Each regimen was tested at 2 energy levels, a low 270 kcal per kilo body weight and day and a 350 which is a hypercaloric level, 350 kcal per kilo and day. We have 64 rats in the beginning, two energy levels, 32 rats each and in each energy level we have a no fat group, low fat group, medium and high fat group.

Let me just go briefly through the animal model. You know the physiology, the biochemistry, the metabolism and the nutritional requirements of the rat are pretty well investigated. There is a lot of experience in most experimental laboratories in the world. Moreover the rat is very small, it's inexpensive, it's very friendly, it's easy to handle so it becomes a very good animal for laboratory, and given its fast growth cycle in its short life span it is what Prof Wretlind calls a living test tube for nutritional studies.

The animals were young animals, weighing about 160 – 170 grams each in the mean, and they were individually housed an adapt to wear a harness, designed to protect a central vein catheter to the back of the rat. After one week adaptation to wear this harness the animals were operated and the silicon catheter was implanted in the superior vena cava through the internal jugular vein and the rats were adapted to one more week to this central vein catheter. After that the experiment started.

The intravenous nurients that were administered to these animals were composed by mixing hypertonic glucose solutions, intralipid 20%, vamin N, distilled water, vitamins and minerals as to complete the requirements for this kind of animal. The nitrogen supply was constant to all the animals, 9 g nitrogen per kilo and day. This is supposed to be enough for the animal, their protein metabolism and to grow and not enough to interfere with glucose or lipid metabolism or at least not interfere too much.

Glucose is given according to this number that you can see here and the triglycerides were 0% in the no fat groups of course, and as it was ratios they are increasing from 1.5 to 2 grams triglycerides per kilo and day in low fat groups, 7.7 and 10.2 in the medium fat groups and 15.3 to 20.4 for the high fat groups. The nutrients were administered. Let me just remind you briefly the composition of intralipid 20%, composed of almost 50% linoleic acid, 7.7 alpha linolenic acid.

The nutrients were administered continuously at a constant rate through infusion pumps during 10 days and after the 10th day the animals were anaesthesised and exsanguinated. Samples were than collected for analysis.

Let us now consider the effect of the different I.V. supplies on the growth. There is a significant difference between all the groups of the high energy level compared to all the groups of the low energy level. So where the animals were fed 350 they did grow better. Control animals were animals orally fed, sham operated and orally fed ad libitum. They were eating approximately 310 and not 350 kcal per kilo and day;

The evolution of the body weight for the low energy level, was studied as the percentage in weight gain. In the very first days, 3 to 4 days, the animals fed no and low fat did lost weight all the other animals were keeping almost no growth in the first days, but there were no striking differences in the weight gain between the different groups. In the high energy level, no group showed loss of weight initially and there are significant difference between the medium fat group as the maximum weight gain for the no fat group which is the lowest one.

The carcass composition of these animals was the following: very stable levels of water at the two energy levels 207, 350 kcal; so water content was pretty stable. The protein content in percentage was higher in the low energy level and lower in the high energy level and the fat content was higher at the high energy level, lower in the low energy level. So it seems that increasing energy to the diet uniformly increases the amount of fat deposition in the carcass and it seems that the different fat to carbohydrate ratios that we can have did not seem to influence so very much the composition of the carcasses. Let us go next to the fatty acid composition of the tissues I have been working with. We have been working epididymal fat, subcutane fat, the tibia's interior muscle and the fat from the liver. Not phospholipids but fatty acid composition of total fat in the liver. The most striking point is that there was almost no differences in the epididymal and subcutane fat. Let us try not to look at polyunsaturated fatty acids, we shall go to there later, let us concentrate on unsaturated and mono-unsaturated fatty acids. There was a tendancy in epididymal fat as well as in subcutane fate which I'll show you later, to keep a stable level of stearic acid and all the others were showing that slight tendency to decrease when the amount of fat in the diets was increased. That you can see also in the subcutane fat. Again you have the stearic acid pretty stable in all the others with a tendency to go down.

Muscle tibialis interior, the saturated fatty acids, the palmitic and stearic acids were pretty stable throughout the experiment, but the palmitic acid showed a steep decrease, either in the low and in the high energy level. You can see that in the low fat high energy level the amount of 16:1 is much higher than at the low energy level this same trend for palmitic acid will be seen later on in the liver. The oleic acid was showing an interesting pattern, it was high in the low fats but higher in the high energy levels and decreasing to a plateau in the low, medium and high fats, regardless of the energy supply.

Considering total fatty acid of liver, the palmitic acid was showing a slight decrease in the high fat groups then it seemed to go down but not with significantly differences. The stearic acid was pretty stable and the palmitic as well as in the muscle we see was going very much down, it was higher in the high energy level compared to the low energy level. Oleic acid shows the same pattern with high levels in the low fat groups especially at the high energy level, increasing to a plateau in the low, medium and high fat groups.

Now we go to analyse what happens with the essential fatty acids in these tissues. Let us start with the epididymal and subcutane fats, since these were the tissues we were less interested things were happening. Linoleic acid was low in the low and medium fat, increasing to the medium and high fat. This was more exaggerated in the no fat group at the high energy level then increasing to a higher plateau maximum levels were reached at the medium and high fat groups at the high energy level as well as in the low energy level. Alpha linolenic were having a tendancy to increase. This was specially observed at the higher energy level where the no fat groups showed the lowest levels of alpha linolenic, in the high fat groups showed the highest levels.

Arachidonic acid was very much stable in epididymal fat. What I said for the epididymal fat is about the same for the subcutane fat. If we go to the muscle tibialis interior the linoleic acid shows also a tendency to get low levels in the no and in the low fat groups in the low energy level reaching to a plateau for the medium and high fat. The same was observed with the lowest levels in low fat at the higher energy groups. Arachidonic acid was normal in the low energy groups but was showed lowest levels at the no fat and in the high fat groups. So they were increasing when more fat was given to the diets in the low and medium and decreasing again when big amounts some 20 grams triglycerides per kilo and day were administered.

The liver linoleic pattern was accentuated what we have been seeing with the tibialis interior. Low levels in the no fat groups, specially when a lot of energy was supplied, it was the lowest level for linoleic acid and tendency to reach a plateau was observed in the medium, in high fat groups, medium and high fat groups. Alpha linolenic was not detected in the no and low fat at both energy levels and was increasing a little bit more in the high energy level than in the low energy level but reaching a plateau in the medium and in the high fat groups. Arachidonic acids were showing more strikingly, what happened with the arachidonic acid, in the muscle at the high energy level and that means low levels for low and high especially at the high energy level with very low levels for the high energy low fat groups in high energy, high fat groups, which were showing the lowest levels observed, so it was increasing to a plateau and then decreasing again when a lot of fat was administered. And again there was one difference between liver and all the others. Finally we were able to detect eicosatrienoic acid, this was high and specially high at the no fat group at the higher energy level, 3.7 as you can see here, 2.0 in the low fat at the low energy level with a steep decrease when fat was added to the animals.

Let me just try to give you not just numbers but the idea of the trends of the acids. Considering linoleic acid in the liver, in the muscle and in the epididymal fat at the low energy level, and also liver, muscle and fat at the high energy level. When we compared liver with liver, we observed a tendency to low levels in the low fat groups for the linoleic acid specially when high energy was supplied to the animals. They were increasing at the low energy, the low fat groups were about the same and the tendancy to reach a plateau which was about the same was observed in the medium and high fat groups regardless of the energy level.

From 7.7 grams to 20 grams of triglycerides per kilo and day you get a plateau and you do not get anymore incorporation of linoleic acid in the liver tissue. In the muscle, the same trend was observed at the low energy level but you can see that the muscle is much more stable. It's probably less influencable by the amount of fat you are giving when you give low energy. At the high energy level, you can see differences, because then the muscle starts incorporating more linoleic acid when you increase, when you give it in the diets. The epididymal fat was shown a relatively stable levels in the low energy levels and increasing levels in the higher energy level, with lower levels in the higher energy level, with lower levels in the low fat groups.

The triene/tetraene ratio that was determined was obviously only in the liver and you can see that although it is not the .4 that was discussed a little bit ago, not even the .2 but there was a striking difference between the triene/tetraene ratios, between the high energy level and the low energy level.

Instead of taking conclusions, I think it's too early in this meeting to take conclusions it's better to discuss. I should say that for growth, the amount of energy is more important than the energy substrate ratio that you administer. For the composition of the different tissues, both energy and the energy substrate ratio have been as shown important. There were no major differences in the two different adipose tissues; the muscles seem to be much more stable than the liver. The liver was the most sensitive organ since it was showing greater variation in fatty acids, variation in arachidonic acid, specially at the higher energy level. It was detectable eicosatrienoic, and the triene/tetraene ratios were observed emphasised with the amount with higher amounts of energy supplies. We should think that fat free regimens induce biochemical imbalances of the fatty acids. Low EFAs in the no and low fat regimens were observed. Eisosatrienoic was present in the liver, again triene/tetraene ratios were detectable and there was observed higher saturated and monounsaturated acids in the no and low fat groups. We have seen that hypercaloric

5

Effect of dietary linoleic, alpha – and gamma – linolenic acids on tissue fatty acids and prostaglandin biosynthesis in animals

Y.-S. HUANG

Efamol Research Institute, Kentville, Nova Scotia, Canada B4N 4H8

Chairman: We will move on to our last session in this morning. Dr Huang from Kentville, Nova Scotia in Canada is giving a paper on "Effects of dietary linoleic, and linolenic acids on tissue fatty acids and prostaglandin biosynthesis in animals."

Dr Huang: Thank you Chairman. I'd like to take this opportunity to thank Dr Ghisolfi and organiser to allow me to participate in this workshop. The title I'm going to present is "Effect of dietary linoleic, alpha – and gamma – linolenic acids on tissue fatty acids and prostaglandin biosynthesis in animals, particularly in rats."

Metabolism of linoleic and alpha-linolenic acids

Linoleic acid (LA, 18:2 n–6) and alpha-linolenic acid (ALA, 18:3 n–3) represent two basic dietary precursors for two different families of essential fatty acids (EFA). The (n–6) fatty acids derived from dietary LA, and the (n–3) fatty acids derived from dietary ALA.

When animals are maintained on diets supplemented with oils rich in linoleic acid, e.g., corn oil, safflower and sufflower seed oils, their tissue lipids become rich in linoleate. Linoleate, cannot be synthesized, but can be metabolized in the animal body through alternate desaturation and chain-elongation to long chain n–6 fatty acids (*figure 1*). Generally, the desaturation of linoleate is regulated by the specific ratelimiting enzymes, delta-6-desaturase (D6D) to form gamma-linolenic acid (GLA, 18:3 n–6) [1]. however, GLA is rarely detected in human or animal

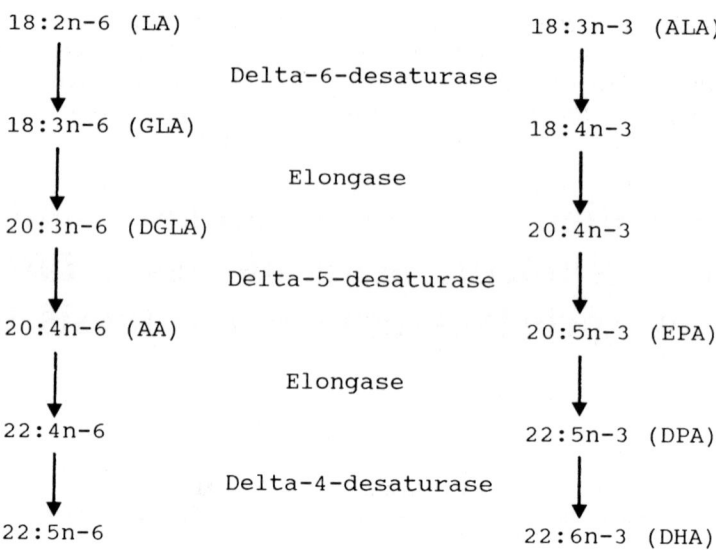

Figure 1. Metabolic pathway of essential fatty acids.

tissue lipids. This is due to its rapid chain elongation to dihomo-gamma-linolenic acid (DGLA, 20:3 n–6) [2]. DGLA is further desaturated by delta-5-desaturase (D5D) to arachidonic acid (AA, 20:4 n–6). AA, in turn, can be elongated to form adrenic acid (22:4 n–6), which is then desaturated by delta-4-desaturase (D4D) to form 22:5 n–6.

ALA, like LA, is metabolized by the same enzyme systems of desaturation and elongation [3]. However, there are competitive interactions between (n–6) and (n–3) fatty acids at various metabolic stages. Evidence has shown that ALA is desaturated faster than LA [4, 5]. The metabolites of ALA, such as eicosapentaenoic acid (EPA, 20:5 n–3) and docosahexaenoic acid (DHA, 22:6 n–3) can exert substantial inhibitory effects on desaturation [6-8], and chain-elongation [9] of (n–6) fatty acids. Thus, excess dietary intake of (n–3) polyunsaturated fatty acids (PUFA) suppresses the metabolism of (n–6) PUFAS, and vice versa [10].

Species differences

Species differences also modulate EFA metabolism. It is known that the activities of various desaturation enzymes vary between different animal species. For example, the cat is deficient in D6D, and thus can not efficiently metabolize the dietary LA [11]. Because of differences in the activities of metabolizing enzymes, the distribution of (n–6) and (n–3) fatty acids in animal tissue lipids varies. In *Table I*, we compared the distribution of (n–3) and (n–6) fatty acids in plasma phospholipids (PL) among different laboratory rodents [12]. The ratios of AA/LA were also cal-

regimens accentuates EFA deficiencies and we have seen that maximal incorporation of EFAs were observed when about 7.7 grams triglycerides per kilo body weight and day were administered to the rats. Thank you for your attention.

Summary

The presence of some fatty acids is essential to maintain normal function of many tissues. The amount and composition of lipid in the diet remains, however, a matter of controversy. Experimental parenteral nutrition may be utilized as a tool to study this problem. An experimental model was designed to investigate the modulating effects of lipids in the fatty acid composition of some tissues.

Normal growing rats were maintained on TPN during 10 days. Four isonitrogenous regimens, differing in the fat/glucose ratio were administered. The fat content was 0%, 6%, 30% or 60% of non protein energy of the otherwise well balanced diets. The infusions were prepared daily using distilled water, hypertonic glucose, Vamin N, Intralipid 20%, vitamins and minerals, and were administered continuously through a central vein catheter, at constant rate. Each regimen was infused at hypocaloric (270Kcal/kg/day) and hypercaloric (350Kcal/kg/day) level, making a total of eight test groups (7-9 animals each). The fatty acid profiles of total liver, muscle and adipose tissues were determined.

The concentration of saturated and monounsaturated fatty acids were higher in the No Fat and Low Fat groups. The amount of EFA (sum of 18:2w6, 18:3w3 and 20:4w6) was lower inthe No Fat groups, particularly at the higher energy level. The triene/tetraene ratio was also increased in the liver tissue of the No Fat groups, more so in the 350 Kcal regimen. Incorporation of EFA in the tissues was generaly maximal in the Medium and High Fat regimens, regardless of the energy level of the intravenous diet. The liver showed more pronounced changes with the different regimens than the muscle while both adipose tissues showed similar and relatively stable fatty acid patterns regardless of the energy level of the regimens.

This study suggests that the requirements of EFA is increased in absolute values when hypercaloric diets are administered.

Discussion

Dr Adam: Thank you Dr Martins for your detailed data on fatty acid distribution in the rat. Who wants to comment on that; it's very interesting all those data showing that special tissues are capable to differentiate the fatty acid uptake, please.

Dr Messing: I want to thank very much Fernando for his excellent work and the point I want to raise is the following: I miss the following point I'm probably you get it. Is the data for your control group; with the same caloric amount, what is the determination of a fatty acids control group?

Dr Martins: We have not determined the fatty acid composition of the control group, this is what we know the rats behave when they are fed and sham operated and fed ad libitum in the laboratory with a pattern of aminoacids and a pattern of diet similar that were administered to the rats. So we do not have any composition of fatty acids of different tissues in these control rats for this experiment.

Chairman: So we do have time for just one more question. Please Dr Ghisolfi.

Prof Ghisolfi: One of the problem to obtain EFA deficiency in rats, is the duration of the protocol period. Why do you choose 10 days and not more?

Dr Martins: Well I think as I told you short life cycle of the rat gives us 10 days as could be comparable to something like 2 to 3 months in a human being. I could think of that and it becomes more difficult to perform parenteral nutrition with good results without dying rats with sepsis you know for much longer than that. We can do this we have done this in the laboratories in Kabivitrum in Stockholm getting rats for almost 45 days in parenteral nutrition but I don't think that anyone can do longer than that.

Chairman: Thank you once more Dr Martins for your detailed data.

culated to reflect the rates of conversion of LA to AA in different animals. Figures in *Table I*, clearly show that different animal species have different levels of conversion activity. Rats can actively convert LA to AA. On the other hand, rabbits and guinea pigs are not as active in converting LA to AA. They are also not very efficient in incorporating the (n–3) fatty acids in plasma PL.

Table I. Fatty acid composition (mg/100 mg total fatty acids) of plasma phospholipids (from [12])

Species	n-6				n-3		
	LA	DGLA	AA	AA/LA	EPA	DPA	DHA
Human	21.5	3.1	11.4	0.53	1.0	0.9	3.5
Rat[a]	18.4	0.9	33.6	1.83	0.5	0.8	6.7
Mouse[a]	26.1	2.3	9.0	0.34	0.9	–	9.8
Hamster[a]	30.0	0.7	7.8	0.26	2.7	0.9	8.3
Guinea Pig[b]	38.0	0.8	7.0	0.18	–	0.6	0.7
Rabbit[b]	43.8	0.1	9.1	0.21	–	–	–

a fed on purina rat chow which contains 4.5% fat (24.3% LA and 3.7% ALA).
b fed on purina guinea pig chow which contains 4% fat (27.1% LA and 3.3% ALA).

Incorporation of linoleic and alpha-linolenic acids

We have also compared the incorporation of LA and ALA in EFA deficient rats. In this study, weanling male rats were first deprived of fat for 8 weeks. The fat deficient animals were then given (600 mg/kg BW) of either LA or ALA ethyl ester by i.p. injection every other day for 10 days. Since plays an important role in the fatty acid synthesis and in the desaturation and chain-elongation of LA and ALA for other tissues [13], liver PL fatty acid profiles, which are shown in *figure 2*, should reflect the metabolic changes of (n–3) and (n–6) fatty acids *in vivo* [14].

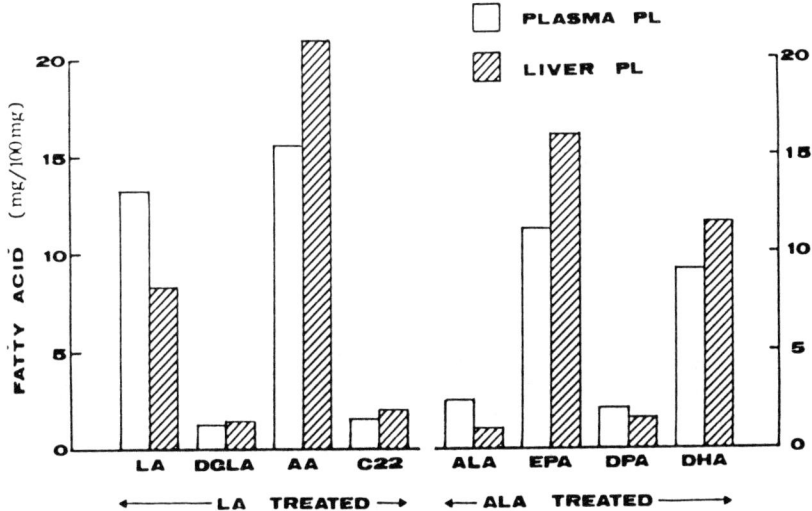

Figure 2. Effect of LA and ALA administration on polyunsaturated n–3 and n–6 fatty acid distribution in plasma and liver phospholipids. (From Huang et al., 1985a).

LA administration significantly elevated the levels of LA and its C-20 metabolite, AA, whereas the administration of ALA did not change the levels of ALA itself, but significantly increased the levels of its C-20 and C-22 metabolites, EPA and DHA. This result indicates that (n–6) and (n–3) fatty acids are not metabolized exactly in the same manner. Earlier, Bernert and Sprecher [2] had demonstrated that AA and EPA can be further elongated to 22:4 n–6 and 22:5 n–3 respectively at a considerable rate. However, long chain (n–6) fatty acid, such as 22:4 n–6, is only abundant in adrenal chlesteryl esters (CE), and 22:5 n–6 in testis PL. Generally, they are minor components in other animal tissues. On the other hand, when ALA is included in the animal diet, the dominant long chain (n–3) fatty acids are EPA and DHA.

As (n–3) and (n–6) fatty acids compete with each other for the same enzyme systems of desaturation and chain elongation, Mohrhauer and Holman [15] have demonstrated that the ratios of dietary (n–6)/(n–3) dictate the tissue fatty acid distribution. We have examined the incorporation rates of (n–6) and (n–3) fatty acid into plasma and liver lipids in EFA deficients rats fed diets with different ratios in LA and ALA in the form of safflower oil and linseed oil (*figure 3*) [16].

Figure 3 shows that PUFAS were favorably incorporated into plasma and liver PL and plasma CE. Correlation between the ratios of (n–6)/(n–3) in diets and those in plasma and liver lipids also demonstrates significant differences in the ratios of (n–6)/(n–3) in plasma and liver lipids in response to dietary ratios (*figure 4*).

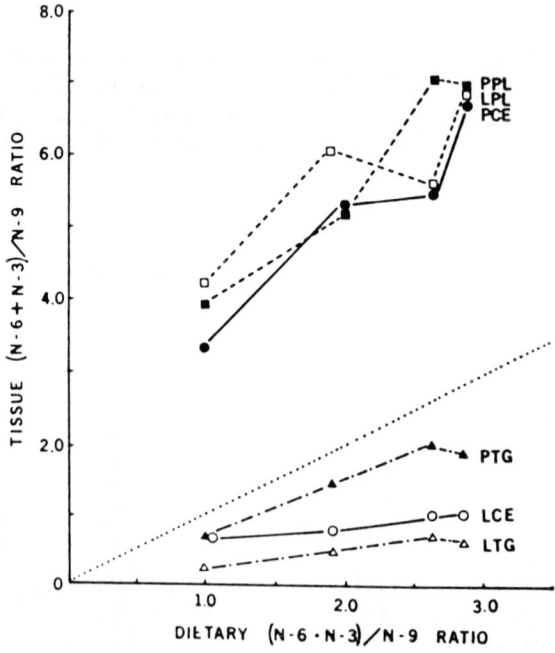

Figure 3. Differential incorporation rate of (n–6) and (n–3) fatty acids into plasma and liver lipids in EFA deficient rats fed diets with different ratios in (n–6) and (n–3 acids. (From Huang *et al.*, 1987).

Effect of dietary linoleic, linolenic acids on tissue fatty acids

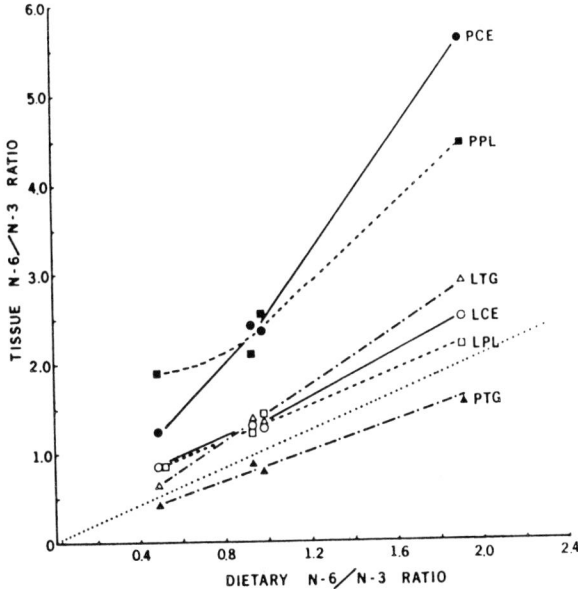

Figure 4. Effect of dietary (n–6)/(n–3) ratios on (n–6)/(n–3) ratios in plasma and liver lipids. (From Huang *et al.*, 1987).

In liver lipids, the (n–6)/(n–3) ratios were neraly on par with those in the diet. On the other hand, the ratios in plasma PL and CE were 2.3 – and 3 – fold of those in the diet. These result (*figures 3 and 4*) indicate a preferential incorporation of (n–6) over (n–3) fatty acids, particularly in plasma PL and CE.

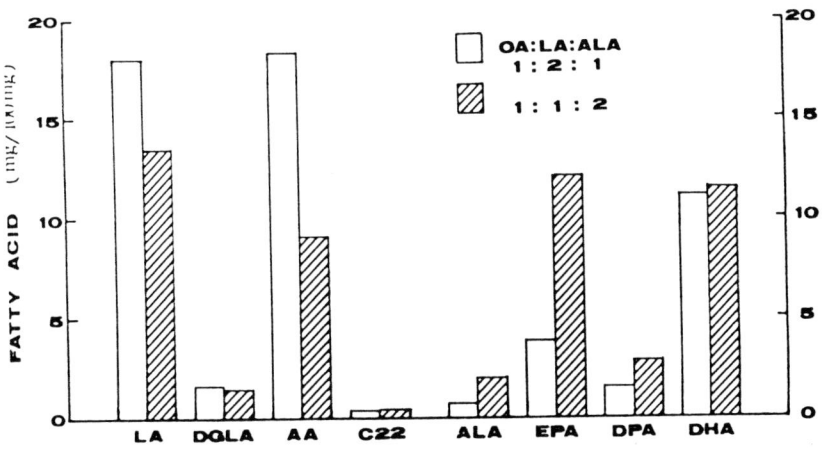

Figure 5. Polyunsaturated (n–3) and (n–6) fatty acid distributions in EFA deficient rats given LA/ALA at ratios of 0.5 and 2. (From Huang *et al.*, 1987).

Essential fatty acids

When animals were given LA/ALA at a ratio of 2 in comparison with that of 0.5, both LA and AA of the (n–6) fatty acids were elevated, but only EPA of (n–3) fatty acids was affected (*figure 5*). It appears that increasing the dietary LA/ALA ratio, elevates LA and AA at the expense of only EPA, suggesting that LA and AA compete with EPA for the same location in PL molecules.

Because oleic acid (OA, 18:1 n–9) also competes with LA and ALA for D6D, the rate-limiting step in eicosanoid synthesis, we have also examined the effects of dietary oleic acid on the liver phospholipid fatty acid profile (*figure 6*).

Figure 6 shows that increasing the dietary levels of oleic acid significantly suppresses the incorporation of (n–6) fatty acids, namely LA and AA, but not of (n–3) fatty acids in liver PL despite the LA/ALA ratio being maintained at the same level. This suggests that oleic acid competes selectively with the position in PL occupied by LA and AA, and that (n–6) fatty acids are more readily replaceable than (n–3) fatty acids by oleic acid.

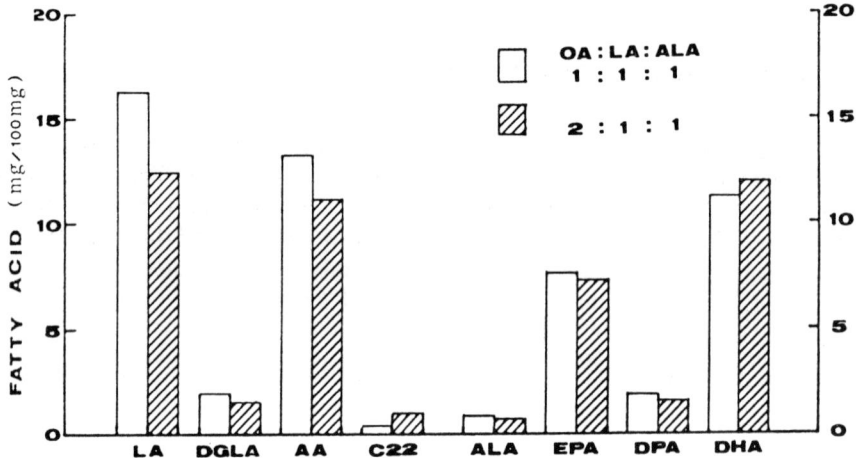

Figure 6. Effect of dietary levels of oleic acid on the incorporation of (n–3) and (n–6) fatty acids in liver phospholipids. (From Huang *et al.*, 1987).

Mechanism responsible for differential metabolism of (n–3) and (n–6) fatty acids

What is the mechanism which causes the differential metabolism of (n–3) and (n–6) fatty acids? Several interpretations have been proposed. It has been suggested that this difference is a result of thehigh specificity of liver microsomal acylglycerophosphorylcholine acyltransferase which synthesizes PL and releases PL into the circulation [17], and of lecithin: cholesterol acyltransferase for plasma CE synthesis [18, 19].

There is another possiblity which may account for the differential incorporation between (n–3) and (n–6) fatty acids. that is the cellular uptake and oxidation rate which varies among different fatty acids by chain length, or the degree of unsaturation. Results in *figure 7* are reported recently by Dr Crawford and his colleagues [20].

Figure 7 shows that the *in vivo* oxidation rate of ALA and OA is faster than that of LA and other long chain (n–6) fatty acids. This difference could, in part, result in the low incorporation of total (n–3) fatty acids in comparison with that of (n–6) fatty acids, as more ALA is diverted to oxidation, less is available for further metabolism.

Hagve, Christophersen and colleagues [21-23] have suggested that the enzymes responsible for elongation and D4D are active with EPA whereas they are less active with AA as substrate. There also exists a preferential retroconversion of C-22 (n–6) fatty acids back to AA [24, 25]. The C-22 (n–6) fatty acids are shortened to C-20 (n–6) acids in the inner mitochondrial membrane or in the peroxisome [24, 26, 27]. These observations would explain the high levels of EPA and DHA in ALA-fed animals, and of AA in LA-fed animals.

Role of GLA in EFA metabolism

The major EFA of the diet is LA. However, LA metabolites, such as GLA, DGLA and AA possess greater EFA activity than does LA itself [28]. The conversion of LA into other (n–6) PUFAS is regulated by a rate-limiting step, delta-6-desaturation [1]. The product of this metabolic reaction is the formation of GLA (*figure 1*). We

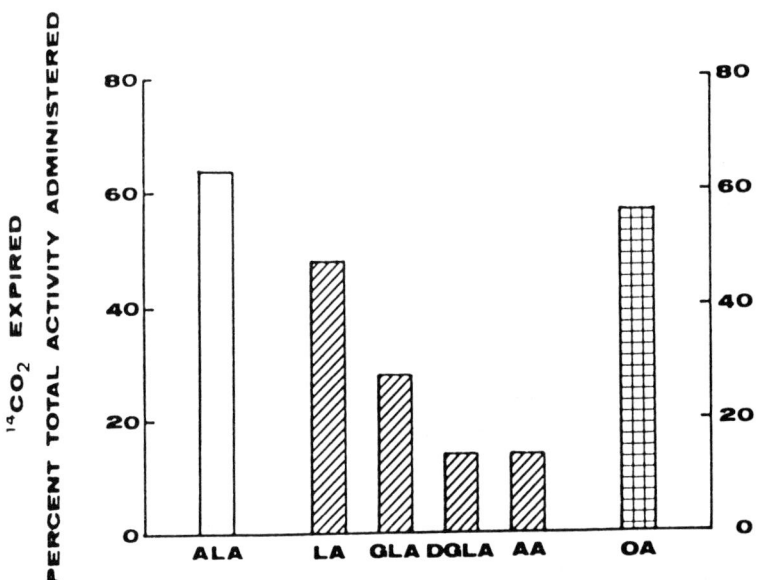

Figure 7. The *in vivo* oxidation rates of ALA, LA, GLA, DGLA, AA and OA in rats (data from Leyton *et al.*, 1987).

have discussed so far, the effect of dietary LA and ALA on tissue lipids. Both LA and ALA are substrates for the rate-regulating D6D. What would be the effect, if D6D product in place of substrate, such as GLA, is supplemented to animals?

Rats in comparison with other speices, are very active in EFA metabolism, and more so when they are in the state of EFA deficiency [29]. Dietary LA in EFA deficient rats can be readily converted into GLA. Under this condition, the formation of AA and other long chain (n–6) fatty acids are not significantly different between GLA-fed and LA-fed rats, with the exception of low levels of LA in GLA-fed rats.

However, there are many nutritional and hormonal factors which interfere with the conversion of LA to GLA [29]. Under the influence of these factors, the ability of animals to convert LA to GLA is significantly reduced. The followings are a few examples which we have observed in our laboratory.

a) *Antioestrogen Tamoxifen* [30]; b) *Diabetes* [31]; c) *Aspirin* [32]; d) *Dexamethasone* [33]; e) *Cholesterol* [34] and f) *Fish Oil Feeding* [8].

All the above mentioned factors directly or indirectly interfere with the conversion of LA to AA (*figure 8*). It is under these conditions that GLA plays a more important role than does LA in EFA metabolism.

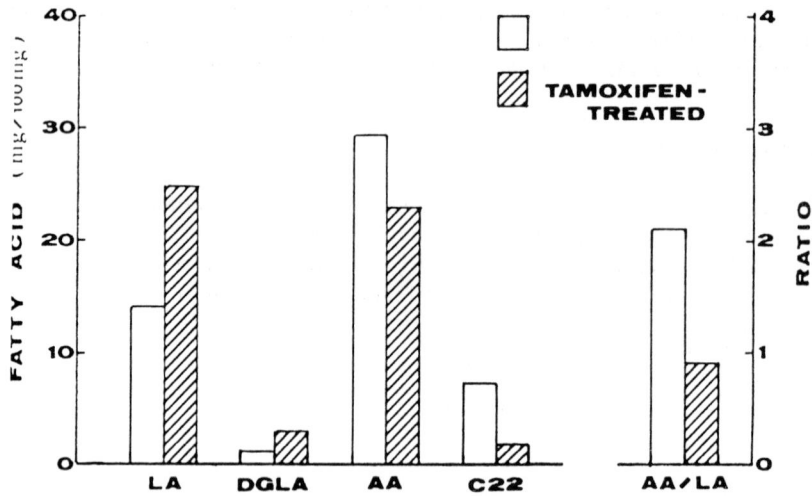

Figure 8. Effect of tamoxifen treatment on the distribution of long chain (n–6) fatty acids in liver phospholipids. (From Huang and Lipton, 1986).

Comparison of the effects between LA and GLA

Diabetes

In experimental and human diabetes, the conversion of LA to GLA is significantly impaired due to the deficienty of insulin. It is believed that the long term adverse effects of diabetes could be caused by inadequate metabolism of LA. Houtsmuller *et al.* [35] treating diabetic patients with high dose of LA could sharply reduce the progression of diabetic micro- and macro-angiopathy. The very high dose of LA used in that trial may have been needed to overcome the defective D6D activity. Indeed, Jamal *et al.* [36] have shown that treatment of diabetic patients with GLA in the form of evening primrose oil significantly improved the symptoms of neuropathy. Chantreuil *et al.* [37] have also shown some improvements in platelet function in insulin-dependent diabetic patients treated with GLA.

Aspirin-induced gastric hemorrhage

It is known that chronic intake of large dose of aspirin induces gastric hemorrhage [38], which could be alleviated by the administration of prostaglandins [39]. The inhibitory effects of aspirin on the formation of AA [32], and on prostaglandin synthesis [40] might be responsible for the development of gastric hemorrhage. In aspirin-treated rats, GLA in place of LA in the diet protected against the aspirin-induced damage [41]. The levels on AA in liver PL were not different in GLA-fed, aspirin-treated or nontreated rats, but were significantly reduced in LA-fed, aspirin-treated rats in comparison with those nontreated rats. Thus, this result indicates that the development of aspirin-induced hemorrhage can be prevented in rats by providing GLA which bypasses the D6D and supplies the substrate for AA formation.

Cholesterol-lowering effect

PUFAS are known to lower plasma cholesterol levels [42]. Since LA metabolites, e.g., GLA and AA, are more effective in cholesterol-lowering than LA itself [43, 44], the hypocholesterolemic effects of LA require the conversion of LA to further metabolites. However, this step is complicated by the inhibitory effect of dietary cholesterol on the conversion of LA to AA [34, 35]. We have demonstrated that dietary cholesterol-induced elevation of plasma cholesterol in animals can be significantly reduced when LA-rich oil is replaced with a GLA-rich oil in the diet (*figure 9*) [34, 46]. This observation has been confirmed by Sugano and his colleagues [47].

Prostaglandin production

AA besides being an important structural components of membrane PL, is also the major precursor of the 2 series prostaglandins (PGs), thromboxanes, and leukotrienes [48]. PGE_1 and PGF_{1a} groups are synthesized from DGLA, whereas PGE_3 and PGF_{3a} are synthesized from EPA. Dietary fatty acids can modify the incorporation and release of fatty acids in the tissue membrane PL, thus, they are important in modulating the prostanoid production and in turn regulating the physiological functions [49].

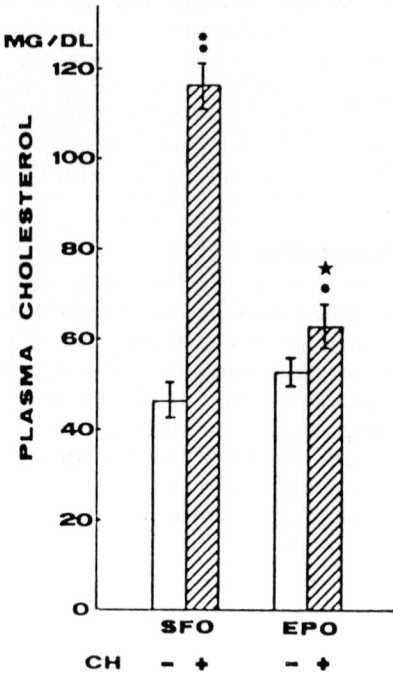

Figure 9. Hypocholesterolemic effect of GLA-rich oil (EPO) in comparison with LA rich oil (SFO) in cholesterolfed or nonfed rats. (From Huang et al., 1984a).

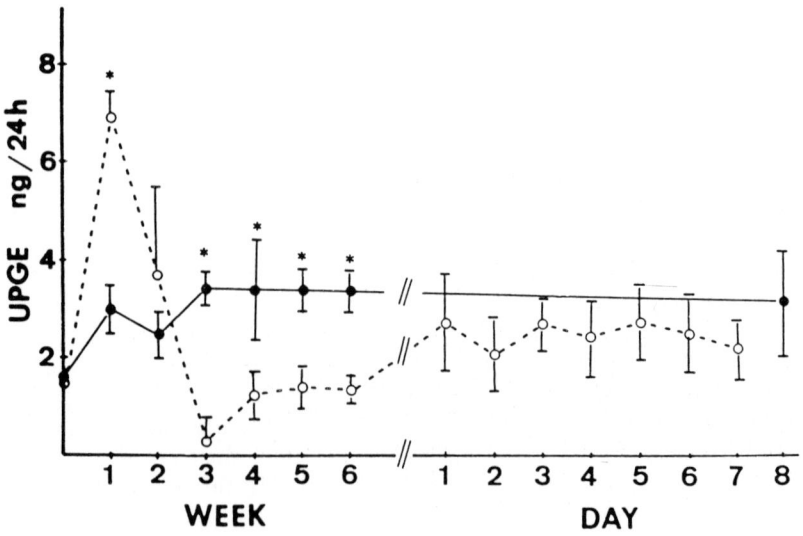

Figure 10. Effect of dietary depletion and repletion of 18:2 n–6 on urinary PGE excretion.

Effect of dietary linoleic, linolenic acids on tissue fatty acids

The availability of AA from LA for PG production

It has been suggested that a constant supply of LA is essential for the biosynthesis of 2 series PGs [50, 51]. The availability of free precursor acids is one of the important factors regulating PG biosynthesis, particularly in EFA deficient rats. In our previous study [52], we placed animals on a EFA-deficient diet for 6 weeks. During the fat deprivation, urinary PGE_2 excretion increased in the first week, but then fell to a low level and remained at that level (*figure 10*). A decrease urinary PGE_2 excretion has also been shown by Hansen [53] in growing rats fed a fat free diet for more than 12 weeks. Within 24 hours of feeding of LA, urinary PGE_2 excretion returned rapidly to normal levels. However AA concentrations in renal PL subfractions remained well below the normal (*figure 11*). [52]. Hansen [53] has also shown that EFA-deficient rats with decreased urinary PGE_2 excretion respond rapidly to a dietary LA supplementation. This raises the question of the source of AA for PG production. It is possible that dietary LA may be rapidly converted to AA and subsequently to PGE_2 without AA levels rising in the lipid fractions [54].

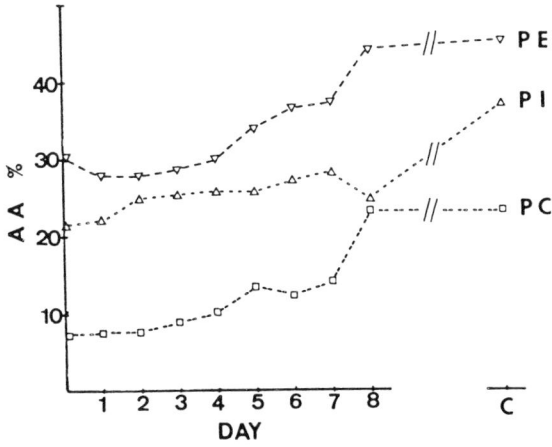

Figure 11. Effect of dietary repletion of 18:2 n–6 on fatty acid composition of various renal phospholipid subclasses.

It has also been demonstrated that a diet rich in ALA depresses rat renal and aortic PG synthesis when compared to a diet rich in LA [55-57]. This is due to competitive inhibition [13] or suppressing the activity of the cyclooxygenase and consequently the synthesis of PGs by ALA itself [58], or its metabolites [6, 59]. *Figure 12* combines data from Mohrhauer and Holman [15] and from Hassam [60], which further illustrates that GLA, in comparison with LA, is more effectively metabolized to long chain (n–6) fatty acids. By by-passing the rate-limiting step, D6D, GLA experiences less degree of competition with ALA when it is supplemented together with ALA in diets to animals.

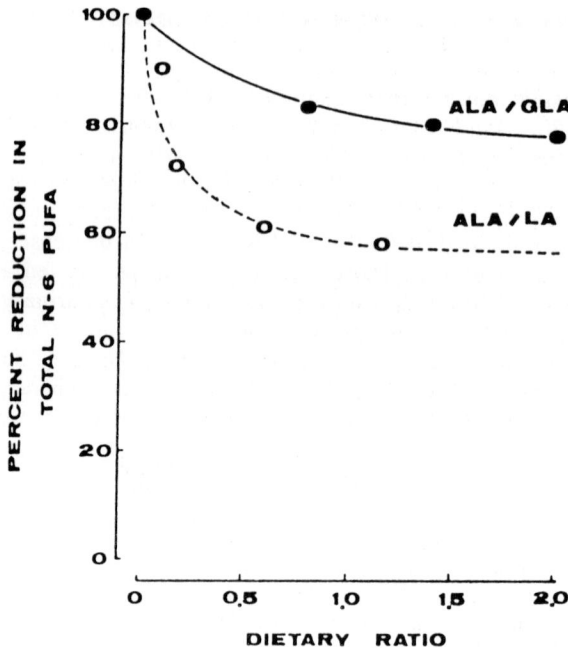

Figure 12. Effect of dietary supplementation of ALA on the metabolism of long chain (n–6) fatty acids in liver lipids. (From Mohrhauer and Holman, 1963 and Hassam, 1977).

In rat PL, DGLA was moderately elevated following intake of GLA [61]. Knapp et al. [62] have demonstrated an increased renal formation of PGE_1 in the rabbit following dietary intake of DGLA.

The result I have presented is in agreement with other reports suggesting that PG production is closely linked to dietary fat intake. However, the results in rats may not be entirely applicable to humans. In animal models, particularly in rats, EFA deficiency enhances the activity of D6D. LA can be readily metabolize to AA and serves as a precursor for PG production. In humans, the presence of various nutritional and hormonal factors, which we have discussed earlier, would significantly hamper the metabolism of LA to AA at the stage of D6D in addition to the fact that humans are genetically low in D6D. The various beneficial effects of GLA in clinical trials could be attributed to its unique characteristic, that is, to bypass the defective D6D step.

References

1. Marcel Y.L., Christiansen K., Holman R.T. (1968) The preferred metabolic pathway from linoleic acid to arachidonic acid in vitro. *Biochim. Biophys. Acta* 164: 25-34.
2. Bernet J.T. jr., Sprecher H. (1975) Studies to determine the role rates of chain elongation and desaturation play in regulating the unsaturated fatty acid composition of rat liver lipids. *Biochim. Biophys. Acta* 398: 354-363.

3. Sprecher H., James A.T. (1979) Biosynthesis of long chain fatty acids in mammalian systems. In: *Geometrical and Positional Fatty Acid Isomers*. Emken E.A., Dultorn H. (eds), pp. 56-90, American Oil Chemists' Society, Champaign, IL.
4. Mead J.F. (1971) The metabolism of the PUFAs. *Prog. Chem. Fats Lipids* 9: 159-192.
5. Brenner R.R. (1981) Nutritional and hormonal factors influencing desaturation of essential fatty acids. *Prog. Lipid Res.* 20: 41-47.
6. Brenner R.R., Peluffo R.O. (1967) Inhibityory effect of docosa-4, 7, 10, 13, 16, 19-hexaenoic acid upon the oxidative desaturation of linoleic into gamma-linolenic acid and alpha-linolenic acid into octadeca-6, 9, 12, 15-tetraenoic acid. *Biochim. Biophys. Acta* 137: 184-186.
7. Nassar B.A., Huang Y.S., Manku M.S., Das U.N., Morse N., Horrobin, D.F. (1987) The influence of dietary manipulation with n-3 and n-6 fatty acids on liver and plasma phospholipid fatty acids in rats. *Lipids* 21: 652-656.
8. Huang Y.S., Nassar B.A., Horrobin D.F. (1987) Changes of plasma lipids and long chain n-3 and n-6 fatty acids in plasma, liver, heart and kdney phospholipids of rats fed variable levels of fish oil with or without cholesterol supplementation. *Biochim. Biophys. Acta* 879: 22-27.
9. Mohrhauer H., Christiansen K., Gan M.V., Deubig M., Holman R.T. (1967) Effect of linolenic acid upon the metabolism of linoleic acid. *J. Nutr.* 81: 67-74.
10. Garcia P.T., Holman R.T. (1965) Competitive inhibitions in the metabolism of polyunsaturated fatty acids studied via the composition of phospholipids, triglycerides and cholesteryl esters of rat tissues. *J. Am. Oil Chem. Soc.* 42: 1137-1141.
11. Hassam A.G., Rivers J.P.W., Crawford M.A. (1977) The failure of the cat to desaturate linoleic acid: its nutritional implications. *Nutr. Metab.* 21: 321-328.
12. Horrobin D.F., Huang Y.S., Cunnane S.C., Manku M.S. (1984) Essential fatty acids in plasma, red blood cells and liver phospholipids in common laboratory animals as compared to humans. *Lipids* 19: 806-811.
13. Brenner R.R. (1974) The oxidative desaturation of an unsaturated fatty acids in mammals. *J. Mol. Cell. Biochem.* 3: 41-47.
14. Huang Y.S., Mitchell J., Manku M.S., Horrobin D.F. (1985) Effect of cholesterol feeding and sex difference on the tissue n-6 and n-3 fatty acid levels in fat-deficient rats treated with linoleate and linolenate. *Nutr. Res.* 5: 535-543.
15. Mohrhauer H., Holman R.T. (1963) The effect of dose levels of EFA upon fatty acid compostion of the rat liver. *J. Lipid Res.* 4: 151-159.
16. Huang Y.S., Hancock R.L., Horrobin D.F. (1987) Selective incorporation of n-3 and n-6 fatty acids in essential fatty acid deficient rats in response to short-term oil feeding. *Biochem. Int.* 14: 659-666.
17. Lands W.E.M., Inoue M., Sugiura Y., Okuyama H. (1982) Selective incorporation of polyunsaturated fatty acids into phosphatidylcholine by rat liver microsomes. *J. Biol. Chem.* 257: 14968-14972.
18. Glomset J.A. (1968) The plasma lecithin: cholesterol acyltransferase reaction. *J. Lipid Res.* 9: 155-167.
19. Sgoutas D.S. (1972) Fatty acid specificity of plasma phosphatidylcholine: cholesterol acyltransferase. *Biochemistry* 11: 293-296.
20. Leyton J., Drury P.J., Crawford M.A. (1987) Differential oxidation of saturated and unsaturated fatty acids in vivo in the rat. *Br. J. Nutr.* 57: 383-393.
21. Hagve T-A., Christophersen B.A. (1984) Effect of dietary fats on arachidonic acid and eicosapentaenoic acid biosynthesis and conversion to C22 fatty acids in isolated rat liver cells. *Biochim. Biophys. Acta* 796: 205-217.
22. Hagve T-A., Christophersen B.A., Dannevig B.H. (1986) Desaturation and chain elongation of essential fatty acids in isolated liver cells from rat and rainbow trout. *Lipids* 21: 202-205.

23. Hagve T-A., Christophersen B.A. (1983) Linolenic acid desaturation and chain elongation and rapid turnover of phospholipid n–3 fatty acids in isolated rat liver cells. *Biochim. Biophys. Acta* 753: 339-349.
24. Hagve T-A., Christophersen B.A. (1986) Evidence for peroxisomal retroconversion of adrenic acid (22:4 (n–6)) and docosahexaenoic acid (22:6 (n–3)) in isolated liver cells. *Biochim. Biophys. Acta* 875: 165-173.
25. Sprecher H. (1967) The total synthesis and metabolism of 7, 10, 13, 16-docosatetraenoic acid in the rat. *Biochim. Biophys. Acta* 144: 296-304.
26. Stoffel W., Ecker W., Assad H., Sprecher H. (1970) Enzymatic studies onthe metabolism of the retroconversion of C22-polyenoic fatty acids to their C20-homologues. Hoppe-Seyler's Z. *Physiol. Chem.* 351: 1545-1554.
27. Bergseth S., Christiansen E.N., Bremer J. (1986) The effect of feeding fish oils, vegetable oils and clofibrate on the ketogenesis from long chain fatty acids in hepatocytes. *Lipids* 21: 508-514.
28. Thomasson H.J. (1962) *Nature* 194: 973.
29. Brenner R.R. (1981) Nutritional and hormonal factors influencing desaturation of essential fatty acids. *Prog. Lipid Res.* 20: 41-47.
30. Huang Y.S., Lipton A. (1986) Effect of the antioestrogen tamoxifen on fatty acid composition of plasma and liver phospholipids in male rats fed n–6 and n–3 polyunsaturated fat enriched diet. *IRCS Med. Sci.* 14: 328-329.
31. Huang Y.S., Fujii K., Takahashi R., Mitchell J., Horrobin D.F. (1985) Effect of diabetes on the metabolism of n–3 and n–6 fatty acids in rats. *IRCS Med. Sci.* 13: 1145-1146.
32. Huang Y.S., Manku M.S., Kent T., Nassar B.A., Horrobin D.F. (1986) A possible new mechanism of action of aspirin and other non-steroidal anti-inflamlmatory drugs (NSAIDs): inhibition of essential fatty acid (EFA) metabolism. *Prog. Lipid Res.* 25: 633-635.
33. Huang Y.S., Das U.N., Horrobin D.F. (1986) Effects of dexamethasone on the distribution of essential fatty acids in plasma and liver phospholipids. *IRCS Med. Sci.* 14: 180-181.
34. Huang Y.S., Manku M.S., Horrobin D.F. (1984) The effects of dietary cholesterol on blood and liver polyunsaturated fatty acids and on plasma cholesterol in rats fed various types of fatty acid diet. *Lipids* 19: 664-672.
35. Houtsmuller A.J., van Hal-Ferwerda J., Zahn K.J., Henkes H.E. (1982) Favorable influences of linoleic acid on the progression of diabetic micro- and macro-angiopathy in adult onset diabetes mellitus. *Prog. Lipid Res.* 20: 377:386.
36. Jamal G.A., Carmichael H. Weir A.I. (1986) Gamma- linolenic acid in diabetic neuropathy. *Lancet* 1: 1098.
37. Chantreuil J., Monnier L., Colette C. et al. (1984) Effect of gamma-linolenate supplementation on serum lipids and platelet function in insulin-dependent diabetic patients. *Human Nutr. Clin. Nutr.* 38C: 121-130.
38. Weiss A., Pitman E.R., Graham E.C. (1961) Aspirin and gastric bleeding. *Am. J. Med.* 31: 266-278.
39. Robert A. (1979) Cytoprotection by prostaglandins. *Gastroenterology* 77: 761-767.
40. Vane J.R. (1971) Inhibition of prostaglandin synthesis as a mechanism of action of aspirin-like drugs. *Nature New Biol.* 231: 232-235.
41. Huang YS., Drummond R., Horrobin D.F. (1987) Protective effect of gamma-linolenic acid on aspirin-induced gastric hemorrhage in rats. *Digestion* 36: 36-41.
42. Kinsell L.W., Partridge J., Boling L., Margens S., Michaels G.P. (1952) Dietary modification of serum cholesterol and phospholipid levels. *J. Clin. Endocr. Metab.* 12: 909-913.
43. Peifer J.J. (1966) Hypocholesterolemic effects induced in the rat by specific types of fatty acid unsaturation. *J. Nutr.* 88: 351-358.
44. Takayasu K., Yoshikawa I. (1971) The influence of exogenous cholesterol on the fatty acid composition of liver lipids in the rats given linoleate and gamma-linolenate. *Lipids* 6: 47-53.

45. Huang Y.S., Horrobin D.F., Manku M.S. (1985) Short-term effect of dietary cholesterol on tissue n–6 fatty acids in fat-deficient rats. *Proc. Soc. Exp. Biol. Med.* 178: 209-214.
46. Huang Y.S., Horrobin D.F. (1987) Effect of dietary cholesterol and polyunsaturated fats on plasma and liver lipids in guinea pigs. *Ann. Nutr. Metab.* 31: 18-28.
47. Sugano M., Ide T., Ishida T., Yoshida K. (1986) Hypocholesterolemic effect of gamma-linolenic acid as evening primrose oil. *Ann. Nutr. Metab.* 30: 289-299.
48. Moncada S., Vane J.R. (1983) Prostaglandins, prostacyclins, thromboxanes and leukotrienes. *Br. Med. Bull.* 39: 290-300.
49. Horrobin D.F., Manku M.S., Huang Y.S. (1984) Effects of essential fatty acids on prostaglandin biosynthesis. *Biomed. Biochim. Acta* 43: S114-S120.
50. Rollner N., Adam. O., Wolfram G. (1979) The influence of linoleic acid intake on the excretion of urinary prostaglandin metabolites. *Res. Exp. Med.* 175: 149-153.
51. Nugteren D.H., Vanevert W.C., Soeting W.J., Spuy J.H. (1980) Effect of different amounts of linoleic acid int he diet on the excretion of urinary prostaglandin metabolites in the rat. *Adv. Prostag. Thromb. Res.* 8: 1793-1796.
52. Huang Y.S., Mitchell J., Jenkins K., Manku M.S. Horrobin D.F. (1984) Effect of dietary depletion and repletion of linoleic acid on renal fatty acid composition and urinary prostaglandin excretion. *Prostaglandins Leukotrienes Med.* 15: 223-228.
53. Hansen H.S. (1981) Essential fatty acid supplemented diet increases renal excretion of prostaglandin E2 and water in essential fatty acid deficient rats. *Lipids* 16: 849-854.
54. Dunham E.W., Balasingam M., Privett O.S., Nickell E.C. (1978) Effects of essential fatty acid deficienty on prostaglandin synthesis and fatty acid composition in rat renal medulla. *Lipids* 13: 892-897.
55. Ten Hoor E.A., de Deckere M., Haddeman E., Hornstra G., Quadt J.F.A. (1980) Dietary manipulation of prostaglandin and thromboxane synthesis in heart, aorta and blood platelet of the rat. *Adv. Prostag. Thromb. Res.* 8: 1771-1778.
56. Hwang D.H., Caroll A.E. (1980) Decreased formation of prostaglandin derived from arachidonic acid by dietary linolenate in rats. *Am. J. Clin. Nutr.* 33: 590-597.
57. Mahoney D., Croft K., Beillin L.J. (1983) Influence of dietary polyunsaturated fatty acids on renal & aortic prostaglandin synthesis in 1 kidney 1 clip Goldblatt hypertensive rats. *Prostaglandins* 26: 479-491.
58. Pace-Asciak C.R., Wolfe L.S. (1968) Inhibition of prostaglandin synthesis by oleic, linoleic and linolenic acids. *Biochim. Biophys. Acta* 152: 784-787.
59. Culp B.R., Titus B.J., Lands W.E.M. (1979) Inhibition of prostaglandin biosynthesis by eicosapentaenoic acid. *Prostaglandins Med.* 3: 269-278.
60. Hassam A.G. (1977) The influence of alpha-linolenic acid (18:3w3) on the metabolism of gamma-linolenic acid (18:3w6) in the rat. *Br; J. Nutr.* 38: 137-140.
61. Hoy C-E., Holmer G., Kaur N., Byrjalsen I., Kirstein D. (1983) Acyl group distribution in tissue lipids of rats fed evening primrose oil (gamma-linolenic plus linoleic acid) or soybean oil (alpha-linolenic plus linoleic acid). *Lipids* 18: 760-771.
62. Knapp H.R., Oezl A., Whorton A.R., Hassam A.G. (1978) Effects of feeding ethyl-dihomo-γ-linolenate on rabbit renomedullary lipid composition and prostaglandin production in vitro. *Lipids* 13: 804-808.

Summary

The phospholipid (PL) fatty acid compositions of cell membranes are modulated by dietary polyunsatured fatty acids (PUFAs) and also by species difference. In essential fatty acid (EFA)-deficient rats, both (n − 3) and (n − 6) PUFAs are selectively incorporated into plasma and liver PL, and plasma cholesteryl esters. There is also a preferential incorporation of (n − 6) over (n − 3) fatty acids. The differential metabolism of (n − 6) and (n − 3) fatty acids could be due to the specificity of enzymes, preferential retroconversion, and differential rates of invivo fatty acid oxidation. Dietary fats also modulate the formation of prostaglandin (PG. In EFA-deficient rats, urinary PGE2 output responds rapidly to a dietary 18:2 (n − 6) supplementation despite the findings that the levels of 20:4 (n − 6), the immediate precursor of PG, in renal PL subfractions were below the normal level. This observation suggests that PG production is closely linked to the availability of 18:2 (n − 6). metabolism of 18:2 (n − 6), particularly the formation of 18:3 (n − 6) − GLA, a delta-6-desaturation product of 18:2 (n − 6) -is subjected to various hormonal and nutritional influences. Evidence has shown that dietary supplementation of GLA, bypassing the impaired D6D, provides some beneficial effects.

Discussion

Dr Adam: Thank you Dr Huang. We should discuss this very important issue on fatty acid metabolism.

Dr Koletzko: You showed this data from very the interesting study of Dr Leyton and co-workers, in London, of the differential oxidation of fatty acids, where omega 6 fatty acids were selectively spared from oxidation when they had higher chain lengths and higher degree of unsaturation such as arachidonic acid. In view of that would you interpret it, interpret the data on the relatively high oxidation of alpha linolenic acid such as alpha linolenic acid has a lower biological value in the rat?

Dr Huang: I wouldn't say that I only suggest that the linoleic acid seems a preferential incorporated in the tissues, that's one interpretation can be because the one alpha linolenic acid uptake into the body is incorporated into the PG first and that can be used for the oxidation in that time. When they start to become long chain polyuinsaturated fatty acids, like EP and DHA then it's a different matter because at that time the oxidation rate tend to be reduced, I say incorporate the phospholipid body not subject to the oxidation as easily as in the PG forms.

Dr Hansen: May I comment on this, you referred to the paper of Leyton and as far as I remember it was radioactive fatty acid skimming to a rat eating a normal rat diet or something like that and of course this rat eats a lot of linoleic acid and compare that with radioactive alpha linolenic acid it's confusing the picture because it has different specific activities so you can't compare the data.

Chairman: It's a very important issue yes of course, let's comment on that.

Dr Koletzko: The results were expressed as per cent activity.

Dr Huang: Of radioactivity yes.

Dr Cunnane: I think it's important point too, I think that actually the human data corroborates that. If you take the studies in which linseed oil has been fed to humans, for instance using as much as 40 g of alphalinolenic acid a day over a period of 4 weeks and has shown that there's no increase in EPA or DHA in the platelets, no in serum phospholipids and I think you have to account for where 40 g of alpha linolenic is going, if it's not going into the longer chain products and it's not substantially increasing itself in those phospholipids, where is it? And I think that the evidence would suggest that there must be a fairly significant oxidation.

Dr Messing: I agree with the previous speakers that oxidation of different type of fatty acid is very important so where are going the phospholipids and my question is: what is the possibility of an accumulation of phospholipid in ther liver according to different ratio of the three series you discuss. You modify your ratio between the three series omega 3, 6 and 9 and you observe a different incorporation of different chain lengths in your phospholipids in the liver and in what group you got the most important accumulation or increase of phospholipid in the liver.

Dr Huang: I probably didn't make my point very clear by talking in a hurry again. If your animals have choice between omega 6 and omega 3, fatty acid tend to be favourably incorporated omega 6 fatty acid according to the results I show. If they have no other choice other than omega 9 compared to omega 6 fatty and this tend to favour omega 6 fatty acid. If they have other choice they always favour the polyunsaturated fatty acid as for omega 6 and omega 3 and between these two omega 6 will be the one favourably incorporated.

Chairman: I think that there could be no doubt that omega 6 fatty acids are more readily incorporated in phospholipids and in other lipids but still there's question not resolved until now. If you are feeding high amounts of alpha linolenic acid the increase of alpha linolenic acid even in adipose tissue is not so big as you should suppose from the level in the diet, and oxidation rates as far as we know the resorption is just the same for linolenic acid as for alpha linolenic acid. This has been shown by liver function studies in man, also in rats and there is until now no idea where to alpha linolenic acid is going and that's a point which is not until now resolved. So are they any other further questions? No, thank you.

6

Regulation of essential fatty acid metabolism during total parenteral nutrition. Nutrient interrelations and particularly interactions of zinc and copper

S.C. CUNNANE

Department of Nutritional Sciences, Faculty of Medicine, University of Toronto, Ontario, Canada M5S 1A8

Chairman: Stephen Cunnane who will talk about "Regulation of essential fatty acid metabolism during total parenteral nutrition. Nutrient interrelations and particularly interarctions of zinc and copper."

Dr Cunnane: Thank you Mr Chairman. Ladies and gentlemen. Prof Ghisolfi I would like to thank you and Kabivitrum for inviting me to come to the meeting. It's a pleasure to come and discuss essential fatty acids and it's a pleasure to be part of the Canadian contingent which I notice is second only to the French contingent amongst the speakers here today and tomorrow. I think that we learnt a lot this morning, at least that we reviewed a lot this morning about the relative importance of omega 6 and omega 3 fatty acids. I think perhaps we raised as many question as we attempted to answer and I'd like to raise the issue and complicate it a little by mentioning that now that we appreciate that there are problems understanding the relative importance of omega 3 and omega 6 fatty acids, we have tod eal with other nutrients as well, because the thesis that I will put to you now or in the next 15-20 minutes is that we can have adequate or optimal amounts of omega 3 and omega 6 and we'll leave aside just exactly what they should be. We can have those amounts present in the diet and we can't necessarily metabolize them as we would wish, and this is the case that I would like to put to you today.

My paper is on the relevance primarily of zinc and copper to EFA metabolism in parenteral nutrition and I'll start at the outset by telling you quite frankly that I have never worked on parenteral nutrition neither in a clinical or an experimental setting, but I believe that there's an important relation between zinc and essential fatty acids which has a very direct bearing on that scenario and perhaps with that foresight that Prof Ghisolfi has asked me to come and talk about it.

Let me put to you the points that are relevant in relation between zinc and parenteral nutrition to start with. First of all in chronic disease, zinc levels are generally lower, whether or not TPN is involved or not. But it doesn't mean that anyone with a low plasma zinc level is zinc deficient or zinc depleted, because depletion of zinc in the plasma is part of a physiological response to trauma, to pregnancy, to infection; it's an acute response and it doesn't indicate that the person is chronically zinc depleted. So that's the first problem. And then as I say zinc depletion is usually present in chronic disease, inflamation and infection, such conditions as would potentially require TPN, so the condition is faced with two issues then of how to deal with those two relevant problems.

The second thing is that if TPN is being given for surgery, we again have as part of the acute response to trauma, which we can call surgery in this context, we again have a depletion of zinc levels. Is this physiological, is it a problem for fatty acid metabolism as chronic zinc depletion is, we don't know.

Again I'm saying to you implicitly in the research that I'm going to present that we may find that the serum essential fatty acid profile in phospholipids particularly may be a better index in fact of zinc status than zinc levels itself or zinc dependant enzymes, and I think we have a case to make in that respect. Implicit in what I'm saying is that zinc is required in essential fatty acid metabolism. Equally I'll address if I have time left the issue of copper and iron.

Let's just look at what zinc deficiency does to just about any species and remark if you will that it's very similar to what Dr Hansen mentioned this morning in relation to EFA deficiency. Slower growth, loss of appetite, skin lesions which are typically ermatitis eczema like lesions, increased water loss across the skin, hair loss and reduced immune response, reproductive sterility in both sexes, impaired parturition, increased perinatal deaths and neonatal mortality and increased capillary fragility from early in the small digits of the feet where there is usually bleeding around the nails, the claws. So these features, this picture of zinc deficienty really essentially mimics that of EFA deficiency and it struck me from when I first learned about that, I felt at that we must learn some more about that connection.

Let me start with a farily classic example and perhaps an extreme example to point out to you what we mean by the relation between zinc and essential fatty acids in a clinical syndrome. AE is acrodermatitis endropathica, very rare disease but it's lethal, and it was only establishabled 15 years ago that there was an acute zinc deficiency that occured through zinc malabsorption and the treatment of these children was very unsuccessful prior to that time. But once it was established that zinc was involved in fact the syndrome has been shown to be virtually purely zinc deficiency. So we start with in this case with someone in 1981 with a plasma zinc level on diagnosis of 7 micrograms per decilitre. There is in this case unquestionably an acute zinc depletion. The sort of depletion you would see with infection would be a drop from 100 to 60 or 70 thereabouts. This is severe zinc deficiency. The pattern of fatty acids taken from that individual in the serum phospholipids at that time show an elevated linoleic at 27 or more % compared to 23 for the controls. Let me skip to arachidonic acid at 6 compared to 11 or 12 in the normal. You'll notice that there's severe depletion of the omega 3s all of them not detectable even the low ones and low levels of 22:6 in comparison with the normal levels. We then go to the stage during repletion two years later when another serum sample is available with a normal zinc level, you'll notice interestingly that linoleic acid is higher than it was and considerably higher than in the controls. But of importance to my discussion is the fact that arachidonic acid is now bounced back from 6 to the normal range of about 12. You'll notice also that the omega 3s are now present and 22:6 is come up from 1 to nearly 3%, very much in the normal range. This person at this time was a teenager and like many of us we will recall are a bit rebellious at that time and would go off zinc on occasion. Only to her detriment and at one particular occasion a few weeks after, well in fact 5 days after this sample her serum zinc is dropped again. You see that the arachidonic acid is heading back downwards again as are the omega 3 fatty acids. This is one case, Dr Koletzko has had cases, Swedes have had cases and we're starting to see a fairly similar pattern of EFAs and serum phospholipids in this disease, indicative of an important effect of zinc on the synthesis primarily of arachidonic acid and I think we can extrapolate and say 22:6 as well although the enzyme data hasn't come in for the omega 3s yet.

Now that's acrodermatitis and that's a rare disease but what I would like to put to you is that there are conditions of considerable relevance to world nutrition such as protein energy malnutrition, which have similarities with acrodermatitis in the way that the fatty acid metabolism is abnormal. Let me show you that. Here we have the control situation, the protein energy malnutrition and then during recovery and this is from Dr Koletzko who's here in the audience. Again I'll be selective in the data I'll show you but you'll see that the linoleic acid levels are similar across the group. So although one would anticipate that in protein energy malnutrition would expect multiple deficiencies, EFA deficiency included in fact the linoleic acid levels in this group of children are similar in all the groups but arachidonic acid is lower in the malnourished children and hasn't in fact recovered at the time that the recovery samples were taken. One also sees that 22:6 is lower and is on its way back. The important thing though is that the triene/tetraene ratio although higher in the malnourished children is not something we would consider as classical of EFA deficiency. And this is the point, here we have essentially similar triene/tetraene ratio across these groups but we find the linoleic acid levels in relation to arachidonic acid the major product are much higher during the condition of malnutrition and have stayed high during the recovery period. So what we have now is a question of metabolic EFA deficiency. These children are not able to either incorporate arachidonic acid but they can synthesize into the serum phospholipids. Whether they can't make it and we can't tell at this stage which it is, but it's not through a deficiency of linoleic acid in their diet or their ability to absorb it. So they are not EFA deficient in the dietary sense and that's what shows up in the triene/tetraene ratio. They have an inability to synthesize the arachidonic acid, triene is as well dependent on the desaturase as is the arachidonic acid. So its synthesis in turn is not increased.

Now, let's go to the experimental evidence to make this point a little clearer. 4 groups of animals, zinc deficient, EFA deficient, zinc supplemented EFA deficient, zinc deficient EFA supplemented and zinc supplemented EFA supplemented i.e the true control situation. So if we're looking for EFA deficient group with normal zinc, and you look for 23 omega 9, in the plasma fatty acids of total lipid profiles, you'll see 23 omega 9 is up there 14%. In the zinc deficients without EFAs it's near 0, as is the true control and it's at the same level in the zinc deficient EFA deficient ones. So when they are EFA deficient 23 omega 9 goes up when they're zinc deficient it doesn't. Yet a lower arachidonic acid level is present in both. Lower arachidonic acid is observed in EFA deficient. In the serum of the rats, in the total lipid profile, we don't see a big decrease in arachidonic acid but the point is that the 23 omega 9 will not go up in a zinc deficient animal although the arachidonic acid synthesis is depressed. This is a study from Brenner's group in La Plata, Argentina, one of the people who has worked the most on the desaturasis and he's been interested in zinc deficiency as well. Let us consider some parts of EFA metabolism, 18:2 to 18:3 which is delta 6 desaturase dependent and 23 to 24 which is delta dependent in control livers, zinc deficient livers, control testis and zinc deficient testis. Delta 6 it drops from 12.5 to 7% conversion and in the testis from 12 to 5 and the delta 5 is dropping from 30% conversion to .7 in liver likewise in the testis from 23% to under 1% with some variability. So both desaturasis 5 and 6 are impaired in zinc deficiency and I think both the composition data and I've only shown you a small selection and the enzyme data would suggest that. But beware because the delta 9 desaturase which is converting palmitic to palmitoleic and stearic to oleic acid is actually elevated inzinc deficient livers.

Now we're seeing a bifurcation in the desaturasis as to the way zinc affects these two and we don't know the basis for it.

What we do know is that schematically the enzyme is sitting in a membrane situation and the terminal desaturasis is part of a group of proteins in which the desaturasis is a terminal component but in fact in order for the desaturase to run the electrons are donated by NADH and through the proteins of cytochrom to the final component. We know that this is an iron containing enzyme the desaturase, so unfortunately the obvious place one would hope that zinc would be involved is not in that particular enzyme although it is a metallic co-factor for a number of important enzymes. In fact it appears from studies also in Canada, but not from my group, that something in zinc deficiency prevents the electron flow from the donor NADH to the desaturase and the impairment appears to be at the cytochrom. So if you are unable to transfert the electrons to the final protein, this in fact would impair the desaturation of that fatty acid and ultimately you have the same effect as if zinc was in fact a component of that enzyme itself.

There's more to zinc deficiency than desaturation. This is another study on acrodermatitis from, I believe, Sweden in which these children were followed, there's two siblings perhaps, I don't recall for sure, followed over a period of eight years. And what they've done here is the triglycerides, cholesterol esters, phospholipids and adipose levels of linoleic acid are shown here over that period of time and over the treatments that were given. You'll notice that up until 1973 quinolone was given as the treatment of choice in acrodermatitis because it was in fact in 1973 that zinc was shown to be a much more effective treatment for it. So this quinoleine was in fact used at that time. Now you'll notice that with this treatment the zinc levels are higher, and decreased without treatment. You'll notice when the zinc intake is high so the linoleic acid levels in these fractions are high and when the zinc drops so does the linoleic acid. Now this data suggests that zinc has a role in the absorption of linoleic acid as well. It may be a weak suggestion from this data. In fact the absorption of long chain fatty acids is in fact dependent on zinc and this, the data is only out for oleic acid, I believe that it would be relevant to linoleic acid as well. A study from a few years ago in which over a period of time you can see that the percentage absorption of trilinoleine, carbon 14 trilinoleine is markedly higher in the controls than in the zinc deficient animals, suggesting that the absorption of long chain fatty acids, oleic specifically in this case, is impaired in zinc deficiency in addition to whatever problem is going on with desaturation. This I think one would consider quite important when you look at TPN for instance given or not total parenteral nutrition but gastric feeding, naso gastric feeding for instance.

So we've talked a little bit about the desaturasis in this particular pathway which you're familiar with now, I'd like to briefly allude to fact that zinc is also involved in phospholipase activity and the net incorporation of long chain fatty acids into phospholipid.

And very briefly in Crohn disease which is probably a disease that will require in some cases TPN, the zinc status is definitely low insome individuals but OK in others. What we did was make a comparison of linoleic acid and arachidonic acid uptake by peripheral blood leukocytes in the low versus the normal zinc ones, and you'll see that the incorporation into phosphatidylcholine and ethanolamine is markedly depressed in those of low zinc status and into phosphatidylcholine by arachidonic acid but interestingly into PE it's little bit higher than in the high zinc ones and what I'm saying to you is basically that we have an additional effect now that's something to do with incorporation, or net incorporation into phospholipids is also affected by zinc status.

Now I'll just skip over that to briefly tell you that in copper deficienty we also have a problem relevant to fatty acid metabolism, essential fatty acid metabolism, but it is not of the same nature as with zinc deficiency. What we find, it is a human experimental study specifically designed to look at experimental copper depletion so it was the only nutrient that was low and it was a good research group doing this, an what they showed was predepletion these were the levels of the four individuals in which we got the data from, so you're following data points consistent with each person. This is 7 weeks depletion at point number one and 11 weeks at point number two, you can see the data as I mention it. This study was shortened from it's originally planned 14 weeks because in the 24 individuals we only got 4 samples.

In the 24 individuals there are 4 myocardial infarctions in this group, in that period within 11 weeks and they had to stop the study. Experimental evidence in copper deficiency, and again if I had more time we could talk about this, shows that arithmias cardiac hypertrophy developing copper deficiency very quickly. I think it's a problem relevant to TPN, you've got to have some copper there.

Now to get back to the fatty acids, you'll see that the arachidonic acid is basically rising over this period time in each individual and the oleic acid is coming down, and 22:6 although it doesn't appear to change much in fact doubles over that period of time. These 2 changes are in fact opposite to what occurs in zinc deficiency. So the metabolism of long chain fatty acids is definitely affected by both zinc and copper and in a way which appears to contrast between the two. The other thing that I think is very important about copper is to realize that the triene/tetraene ratio is also a red herring in relation to copper for the reason that you'll get the triene formed 23 N – 9 with copper supplementation. Because copper stimulates the delta 9 desaturase and producing more oleic acid in turn whether through competition of further stimulation, allowing 23 omega 9 to be synthesized in an apparently healthy adequately nourished series of rats. If we're looking at the control animals here, the low copper animals, their oleic acid is dropping, compared to control animals in liver, plasma, heart. In the copper supplemented ones, the oleic acid is more than double in the plasma, it's elevated but certainly not double in the liver and also marginally elevated in the heart and now you have the appearance of 23 omega 9. So be careful when you decide what the EFA status of an individual is based on a triene/tetraene ratio, with both zinc and copper causing some interfering effects on it.

And I'll finish up with a very brief mention of iron to add to your woes. I've looked at iron deficiency because desaturasis are iron containing enzymes, so how important is this dietary iron intake when you consider that worldwide it's the biggest single nutritional problem that we face. And we see now a classical situation, it's serum phospholipids, polyunsaturated fatty acids, linoleic acid at 18 in the deficient compared to 13 in the controls, arachidonic acid marginally down at 17 from 20, 21. 22:6 I've stuck on the bottom here 5 and .7 I don't see a difference there. But I think that there is something to keep in mind about iron as well in relation to the synthesis of arachidonic acid, there's a lot more work to do on iron so I can't say that this is necessarily going to stand up in a clinical situation but it's something to be aware of.

So to conclude let's just remember that zinc, copper and iron are obligatory for optimal EFA metabolism. You can have adequate EFA in a diet or in your preparation, if the zinc, copper and iron are not there in adequate amounts you won't get them metabolized in the way you would wish. Zinc status can be a significant problem in conditions requiring TPN and EFA profiles may in fact be useful to indicate both abnormal EFA status as wall as zinc status. Finally we need to monitor both the zinc, copper and iron status as well as the EFA profiles in TPN. Thank you very much.

Summary

Among the nutrients demonstrated to be required for adequate essential fatty acid metabolism, zinc is probably the one most affected by the catabolic state frequently present in individuals requiring total parenteral nutrition (TPN). Any physiological or metabolic stress affects blood zinc levels through a mechanism thought to involve release of interleukin 1 which mobilizes zinc from the circulation to the liver where it is incorporated into metallothionein. Acute stress has this effect temporarily and is of little consequence to zinc status in the well-nourished individual. Chronic infection, inflammation or major surgery, especially in the growing infant may seriously impair zinc status because periods of rapid growth are when zinc is required most. Zinc is the nutrient which is best known to affect essential fatty acid (EFA) metabolism. Studies over the past ten years have clearly shown that zinc is required for the desaturation of linoleic acid (18:2 n − 6) and probably alphalinolenic acid (18:3 n − 3). Consequently, the synthesis of arachidonic acid (20:4 n − 6) and probably docosahexaenoic acid (22:6 n − 3) is acutely dependent on zinc status. Zinc deficiency therefore causes metabolic EFA deficiency even in the presence of adequate intake of linoleic acid. The biochemical assessment of EFA status in zinc deficiency is a particular problem in light of the fact that low zinc status will prevent the appearance of the fatty acid which typifies FFA deficiency, namely, eicosatrienoic acid (20:3 n − 9) the synthesis of which depends on the desaturase-elongase pathway. The ratio of 18:2 n − 6/20:4 n − 6 is currently the best marker of zinc status in relation to EFA metabolism. In view of the lack of known storage sites for zinc in the body, it is evident that successful management of the essential fatty acid status of patients on TPN requires close attention to zinc status. Nevertheless, normal EFA profiles in plasma are restored rapidly with zinc supplementation. Other nutrients of importance to maintaining normal FFA metabolism include iron (present in the desaturase protein), copper and vitamin E. iron deficiency also impairs arachidonic acid synthesis while copper deficiency is associated with higher levels of highly unsaturated fatty acids. Copper excess stimulates production of oleic acid (18:1 n − 9) and 20:3 n − 9. Since copper interacts acutely with zinc there by affecting EFA metabolism, the balance between the dietary intake of these two metals is a critical determinant of EFA status.

Discussion

Dr Bourre: Yes I think your lecture makes it more complicated, all of it. Now it's open to questions, yes?

Prof Navarro: My question is about biological signal of cystic fibrosis and zinc status. Some cases are difficult to interpret because we have also FA deficiency, in some cases zinc deficiency and perhaps also vitamin E deficiency.

Dr Cunnane: Well I had space to put it in the abstract but not time to elaborate it. I wanted to make sure that the zinc came across clearly and to leave some of the less well-known nutrients such as vitamin E in relation to the desaturase process out of it. I can't answer specifically what vitamin E is doing as an anti-oxidant. There's a lot of work which has been done on it and I haven't done any. But I can tell you vitamin E is also important in arachidonic acid synthesis as well as whatever antioxidant and peroxidation process it may be protecting against. Our experiences from a couple of years ago was that vitamin E supplementation was in fact reducing synthesis of arachidonic acid and elevating the levels of the precursor dihomogamma, which might be of interest to people who want to increase the 1 series prostaglandins for instance to reduce platelet aggregation, produce information etc. So there's a useful semi-pharmacological role of vitamin E there that may not be related to its anti-oxidant process at all. Of course desaturation is a process of oxidation in fact anyway, so perhaps that's synonymous. Vitamin A, Dr Huang, you've studied vitamin A, I don't know whether we can say conclusively what vitamin A is doing in relation to the EFA metabolism and it's certainly true that it has an important connection with zinc. But I really can't tell you the significance for TPN or even for clinic significance in relation to fatty acid metabolism.

Dr Bjerve: Yes, I just want to ask you: What do you think about the possibility that copper and zinc act both on different enzymes through a same mechanism which means that on the one hand you have enchanced mono-unsaturated fatty acids and on the other hand controlling the polyunsaturated fatty acids – and what about the level of the enzymatic activities and what about the role of these metals on the enzymes – and related to the tocopherol and vitamin E, vitamin E can control to a certain extent the enzymatic activity directly not through peroxidation so may be it is the same story, in fact, in the enzyme?

Dr Cunnane: I think, like many of us, that we're on the tip of an iceberg with this and are just looking down and seeing what there is underneath. I, when I first started studying zinc, I realised the connection between the antagonistic or inverse connection between zinc and copper and married many biological systems. And here we see a classical inverse relationship in relation to the long chain fatty acids, one pushing through the monounsaturates the other important for the polyunsaturates. I can't tell whether that connection is in fact controlling that pathway but there's obviously something that needs more work on. I've done very little enzyme work to explore it more. The whole thing is just begging for some more work.

Dr Bjerve: You mentioned on your last slide that you could use EFA profiling for establishing whether you have a zinc deficient patient or a copper deficient patient. Would it be possible at all to evaluate one set of data from a patient where you don't know the supply of calories, the supply of EFA or do you imply that if you know the patient will have a sufficient intake of EFA then you can use the fatty acid profiling or can you use a fatty acid profiling also in the presence of low intake of EFAs?

Dr Cunnane: Well, you can take certain information and make a guess and if it's an educated guess because you have some background information then the chances of being correct through go up higher. You shouldn't see an elevated 23 omega 9 in zinc deficiency and I don't think anyone has reported that you will. So if you have a patient with symptoms of dermatitis and so on, loss of appetite and weight loss or a child that's not growing, so you say: well, what's the problem? 23 omega 9 is not up, it shouldn't be dietary EFA deficiency. But if the symptons are there perhaps zinc is involved specially if arachidonic acid is low. The same with copper if arachidonic acid is not low but 23 omega 9 is there you can only guess that maybe copper is involved. My data is there's a few people doing some work but it's hard to extrapolate from one or two papers and say yes the whole clinical spectrum now we can figure it out, but we have the profiles, we're starting to see unique patterns causing deficiency for copper deficiency, for EFA deficiency and when you combine EFA and zinc deficiency we don't see a raise 23 omega 9 and I think this has been baffling a lot of people doing clinical work on EFAs. Why is 23 omega 9 not up? Is it because the desaturase is not working even though in EFA deficiency the desaturase should be quicker? Or is there some interference preventing its synthesis as in zinc deficiency? So these are just clues and they are just the start but I think it is going to help us and we take the case which Dr Koletsko and I worked on, we in fact find change in the fatty acid pattern typical of zinc depletion without seeing a change in the plasma levels of zinc. So now we've got perhaps something better indicative of zinc status than zinc itself.

Dr Adam: I think it's very important the way and what you're trying to do it trying to get definite criteria for establishing when you have EFA deficiency, because the only thing we have is this Holman ratio and Holman changed this ratio himself and the data it's built on that could be better seen from a clinical standpoint.

Dr Cunnane: Certainly, I think that the foundations that Holman has helped develop for us.

Dr Adam: I'm not complaining but it means it has to be worked on further. I have one other question – You said, it's much more difficult to analyse serumphospholipids than total serum lipids. Do you need the phospholipids or can you get same information from total plasma lipid?

Dr Cunnane: No way, you have to have the phospholipids an I'll talk to you about this afterwards or anyone who wants to discuss this. The response of the triglyceride pool is much more variable and what goes up and down in triglyceride is palmitic, oleic and linoleic acid. Arachidonc acid in fact stays low so that if triglyceride is elevated arachidonic acid is depressed proportionally, quantitatively it is quite stable and that's another issue. So in the reverse situation in starvation when triglyceride is low arachidonic acid proportionally will be high, that doesn't happen in phospholipids, phospholipids quantitatively are pretty stable. So you've got to look at the phospholipid pattern and regardless of the technical problems which I don't think are hard to overcome, in fact one should restrict it to the phospholipids to interpret this sort of data and it's the one reason why the rat study in which the total plasma profile showed a very weak effect on arachidonic acid, because the triglyceride levels are depressed and a proportional composition of arachidonic acid is up in serum triglycerides and zinc deficient rat so you negate the effect on arachidonic acid levels.

Dr Messing: In patients where the chronic inflamation we find a depressed iron in serum and all signs of iron deficiency and couldn't it be the same way in the states of copper or zinc deficiency and mustn't you be aware of the status of the patient to define conclusions from the deficiency?

Dr Cunnane: One sample, it will not be enough, I think, at all and the important thing with zinc deficiency is to establish what effect supplementation has because in an acutely zinc depleted person in trauma or infection zinc supplementation will not change their condition because they are going to recover and be all right anyway, but in a chronically zinc depleted individual there will be an effect on the fatty acid pattern and on the clinical status, so you can't pick one slice of time and say I know something, you can only say I've got something to look for now.

Dr Messing: So you give very nice information concerning the modification of the levels of different metabolite of fatty acid elongation but have you made measurements of enzyme activity, I understand not?

Dr Cunnane: I've shown you some here, half way through Brenner is the desaturase work, on delta 5 and 6, in liver and testis, and it has been done by a number of people, I haven't specialized in that.

Dr Messing: And the next step is, have you any physiological modifications according modification of production, for example, for arachidonic acid concerning prostaglandin production?

Dr Cunnane: In general in zinc deficiency prostaglandin production is increased from a variety of studies, it's not related to the amount of arachidonic acid synthesis it's related to zinc's anti-oxidant effects in membranes by itself. And any time you have a perturbation of the membrane whether it's physical, chemical, metabolic you're going to increase prostaglandin production and this in fact is what occurs in zinc deficiency.

M. Lindholm: There are many reports on the literature that essential fatty acid pattern in plasma does not really reflect the fatty acid pattern in the membranes and that maybe is the most important part. Do you really think that it's relevant to measure the fatty acid pattern in plasma or shall we measure in some other compartment?

Dr Cunnane: Well first of all what choice do we have, we can certainly look at red cells. If you take red cells you've got to wash them, you may stimulate them to have phospholipase activity so you've got a series of problems to deal with, but I agree membrane composition and serum phospholipid or lipoprotein composition are not necessarily the same. This is only a marker and an index, but a thing is if the rat studies show the defects on the testis, heart, liver are similarly reflected by the serum composition, so I think we're seeing parallels between clinical or experimental status and this profile and I do agree that serum is not necessarily a reflection of membrane activity but there appears to be a correlation or a relevance of that data to the clinical status whether it's acrodermatitis or not Crohn disease or a number of others so I think we've got something to work with.

Essential fatty acids and total parenteral nutrition.
Ed. J. Ghisolfi, John Libbey Eurotext, Paris © 1990, PP. 81-93.

7

Linoleic acid intake and prostaglandin formation

O. ADAM

Medizinische Poliklinik der LMU Pettenkoferstrasse 8a D-8000 München 2, Federal Republic of Germany

Introduction

The incorporation of polyunsaturated fatty acids with 20 carbon atoms in body cells is determined by their dietary intake and by their biosynthesis from linoleic and alpha-linolenic acids. We investigated the incorporation and metabolism of these two parent fatty acids in man with liquid formula diets (LFD), providing a constant amount of linoleic and alpha-linolenic acids over the experimental period, to investigate the competition for incorporation in plasma lipids. With this experimental design the metabolism of linoleic and alphalinolenic acids can be evaluated in man [1], if the LFD are devoid of arachidonic and eicosapentaenoic (EPA) acids.

If the effect of dietary polyunsaturated fatty acids on prostaglandin (PG)-biosynthesis is to be measured, this only can be done with LFD, because a multitude of nutritional factors are known to alter PG-biosynthesis. Beside n–3 fatty acids, which are found indifferent amounts in vegetable nutrients, also vitamine B_{12}, E, and C, pyridoxine, pantothenic acid, riboflavins and biotin are active [2-5]. With conventional diet the intake of these compounds is unpredictable and the effect of one fatty acid in the diet cannot be evaluated. Moreover determinations of PG-biosynthesis should be done in females, because in males unpredictable amounts of prostaglandins, derived from the genital tract, may contibute to PG-formation.

Abbreviations used
- EPA : eicosapentaenoic acid (20: 5, n-3)
- HDL : high density lipiproteins (d>1.063)
- LDL : low density lipoproteins (d 1.006-1.063)
- LFD : liquid formula diets
- PG : prostaglandin

Effects of linoleic acid intake on plasma lipid levels and on arachidonic acid formation

Linoleic acid intake increases the percentage of linoleic acid in plasma lipids and lowers simultaneously plasma lipid levels [6]. The latter effect limits the amout of linoleic acid, which can be transported in plasma lipids. Our studies on this subject revealed a surprising similarity in the changes of cholesterol and phospholipid values. The ratio of these two plasma lipids was constant during nine different amounts of linoleic acid intake, furthermore it became clear, that lecithin was responsable for the changes of phospholipids [6]. In vivo phosphatidyl-choline (lecithin) and phosphatidyl-inositol are the assumed precursor pools in membrane phospholipids, but also minor phospholipid fractions may contribute to PG-formation [7-9]. In cell culture studies the availability of precursor substances is the rate limiting step for PG-formation [3]. Thus, the concentration of lecithin as well as the amount of linoleic acid present is of importance for the availability of linoleic acid for PG-formation.

Metabolic studies showed that LDL transport phospholipids to peripheral tissues and that HDL are concerned with the centripedal transport to the liver [10]. To get a better understanding of the sequellae of linoleic acid supply for PG-precursor availability, the fatty acid pattern of lecithin in LDL and HDL was determined. Experimental subjects were six healthy females being given LFDs, providing a linoleic acid intake of 0%, 4% and 20% of energy intake. These LFDs were given to the experimental subjects for 2 weeks each, always two persons starting with one of the LFDs in a different order. Fatty acids were determined at the end of each two

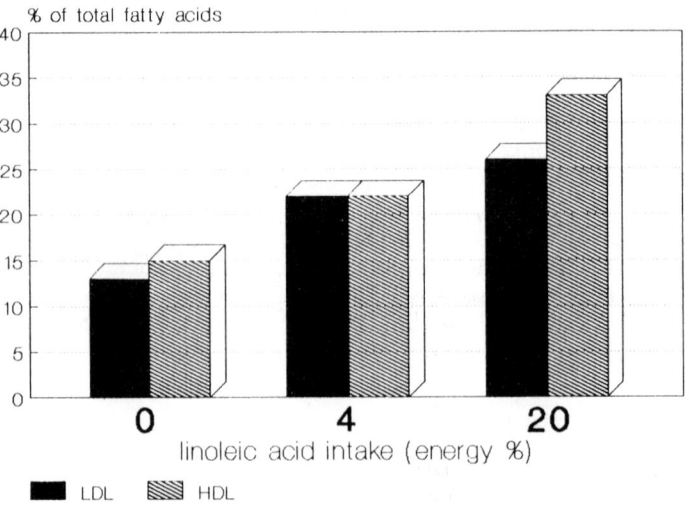

Figure 1. Percentage of linoleic acid in phosphatidyl-choline of LDL and HDL in six healthy females (age 23-32 years) at the end of two weeks of LFD providing a linoleic acid intake of 0, 4 and 20 energy%.

weeks LFD period by gaschromatography, and their quantitation was achieved by calculating the percentage of the fatty acid content in the individual lipid.

At the end of the LFD devoid of linoleic acid all subjects demonstrated the lowest linoleic acid content in the lecithin of LDL and HDL. The data of the period with 4 energy% linoleic acid intake showed the expected increase in the percentage of linoleic acid present, which was similar in both lipids. At the end of the LFD providing 20 energy% linoleic acid, the increase of linoleic acid in HDL was greater than in LDL (*figure 1*). Quantitation of the amount of linoleic acid of the average present in LDL lecithin, showed a decrease with a linoleic acid intake of 20 energy%, compared to the values at the end of the LFD period with 4 energy% linoleic acid intake. This decrease was traceable to the reduction of LDL lecithin in the plasma, while the absolute amount of linoleic acid in HDL lecithin increased slightly [6]. As LFD werde devoid of arachidonic acid, neither the percentage nor the absolute amount of this fatty acid changed in LDL lecithin under these experimental conditions. In contrast, the percentage as well as the absolute amount of arachidonic acid in HDL lecithin decreased with high linoleic acid intake (*figure 2*). This observation is compatible with a reduced activity of desaturating enzymes in the liver, and in peripheral tissues, which transform linoleic acid to arachidonic acid. A decreased activity of the metabolizing enzyme, the delta-6-desaturase, by polyenoic acid intake, has been reported in vitro and in cell culture studies [11].

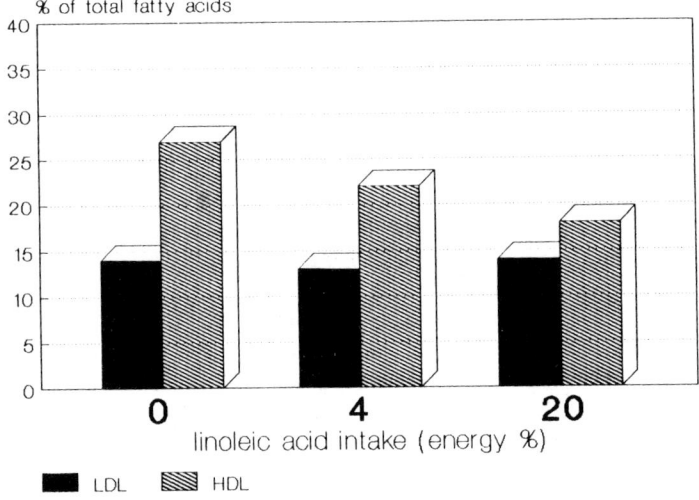

Figure 2. Percentage of arachidonic acid in phosphatidyl-choline of LDL and HDL in six healthy females (age 23-32 years) at the end of two weeks of LFD providing a linoleic acid intake of 0, 4 and 20 energy%.

Effect of alpha-linolenic acid intake on linoleic acid incorporation and metabolism

Alpha-linolenic acid, like other n–3 fatty acids, is bound to the metabolizing enzymes, e.g. delta-6-desaturase, preferentially to linoleic acid [12]. If this enzyme is inhibited by alpha-linolenic acid, a diminished formation of arachidonic acid can be observed. The decrease of arachidonic acid is measurable, as shown above, in the lecithin of HDL and plasma cholesterol esters, if no arachidonic acid is provided with the diet. Contrasting to the findings in vitro, experiments in humans on conventional diet, containing arachidonic acid, had shown no depression of arachidonic acid levels in plasma lipids, even if high amounts of alpha-linolenic acid were given. We decided to reanalyze this subject with LFD, devoid of arachidonic acid in females aged 25-32 years.

The composition of all LFD was identical, with the exception of the composition of the fat. Protein provided 15%, carbohydrates 55%, given as oligopolymeres of glucose, and fat 30% of total energy intake. The LFD were given to each two experimental subjects in a different order. The dietary fat contained a constant amount of 4 energy% linoleic acid and an alpha-linolenic acid intake of 0, 4, 8, 12 or 16 energy was given for two weeks each. At the end of each two weeks period fatty acids in plasma cholesterol-esters were determined. Linoleic acid was not replaced by alpha-linolenic acid in plasma-cholesterolesters. On the contrary, with an alpha-linolenic acid intake of 12 or 16 energy even a small increase of linoleic acid could be observed, indicating a diminished utilisation of linoleic acid [13]. This assumption was confirmed by the determination of arachidonic acid. Arachidonic acid in cholesterol esters decreased with an alpha-linolenic acid supply of more than 12 energy%. This finding indicates that a high intake of alpha-linolenic acid inhibits the desaturating system, which transforms linoleic acid to arachidonic acid. Weiner [14] showed in rat kidney cell culture studies that in vitro the inhibition of arachidonic acid formation by n–3 fatty acids is dependent on the amount of alpha-linolenic acid present in the medium. In our experiment an increase of EPA by 1.6% was noted in plasma lipid with an alpha-linolenic acid intake of 16 energy%. As dietary EPA readily replaces arachidonic acid in nutrition experiments [15], it cannot be excluded that also endogenous formed EPA is responsible for the decrease of arachidonic acid. Taken together, the inhibitory effect of alpha-linoleic acid on linoleic acid metabolism in humans is very small.

Alpha-linolenic acid incorporation in plasma cholesterol esters was low. Even with a dietary supply of 16 energy% alpha-linolenic acid accumulated to only 7% of the total plasma cholesterol fatty acids. Compared to the percentage of linoleic acid, which was 53%, and taken into account that linoleic acids supply with this formula diet was only 4 energy%, the incorporation of linoleic acid in plasma cholesterol esters was about 30-fold that of alpha-linolenic acid. EPA, which was not provided with the diet, increased to 1.6% of total fatty acids in cholesterol-esters with an alpha-linolenic acid supply of 16 energy%. In these experiments we fond a relationship of alpha-linoleic acid to EPA of 7:1 in the fatty acids of cholesterol-esters (*figure 5*), indicating that 14% of the alpha-linolenic acid, incorporated into cholesterol-esters had been converted to EPA [15].

These results indicate a preferential incorporation of linoleic to alpha-linolenic acid into plasma lipids. This was confirmed by another study, in which alpha-linolenic acid was given in a constant amount of 8 energy% with LFD, while the intake of linoleic acid was increased from 0 to 1.7 and 4 energy%. For comparison purposes a formula diet devoid of polyunsaturated fatty acids indexed 0/0 and one formula diet without linolenic acid indexed 4/0, was included. After two weeks on each LFD linoleic acid was incorporated according to the dietary supply. Again no depression of linoleic acid levels was found with increased alpha-linolenic acid intake. On the other hand the percentage of alpha-linolenic acid in plasma cholesterol esters decreased with augmented linoleic acid intake (figure 3). This results also indicates a preferencial incorporation of linoleic compared to alpha-linolenic acid into plasma cholesterol esters and, furthermore, it showes that alpha-linolenic acid incorporation into plasma cholesterol-esters is dependent on linoleic acid intake.

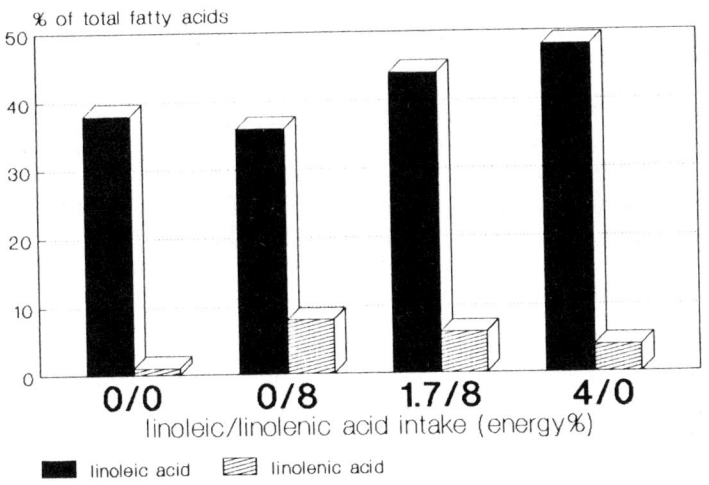

Figure 3. Effect of dietary linoleic acid on alpha-linolenic acid incorporation into plasma cholesterol-ester during an alpha-linolenic acid intake of 8 energy%. For comparison a LFD without essential fatty acids (0/0) and without alpha-linolenic acid (4/0) was given.

Our results have been obtained in short-term experiments may show some differences, because the activity of the metabolizing enzymes, especially the delta-6-desaturase and the cyclo-oxygenase, seem to be regulated by long-term dietary habits. Dyerberg et al. [16] and Bronsgeest-Schoute et al. [17] measured the percentage of linoleic acid, 18:2, n–6, arachidonic acid 20:4, n–6 and EPA 20:5, n–3 in eskimos and caucasians on different diets. Eskimos on their traditional sea-food diet have a lower percentage of linoleic acid in plasma phospholipids than caucasians. If eskimos were put on a western diet, the percentage of linoleic acid surpassed the values, found in caucasians on an eskimo diet, indicating a diminished utilisation of linoleic acid. This was confirmed by the measurements of arachidonic acid. Eskimos on western diet show less arachidonic acid in plasma lipids, compared tocaucasians (figure 4). From this it was concluded that desaturating enzymes in eskimos are less active than in caucasians, leading to a decreased formation of arachidonic acid. If on the other hand caucasians were put on an eskimo-diet the concentration of arachidonic acid is higher than found in eskimos. This finding indicates a long-term dietary regulation of the delta-6-desaturating enzyme. Because the incidence of coronary heart disease in eskimos on a western diet becomes as frequent as seen in caucasians [18], the role of delta-6-desaturating enzyme and the resulting formation of arachidonic acid on atherogenesis needs further evaluation.

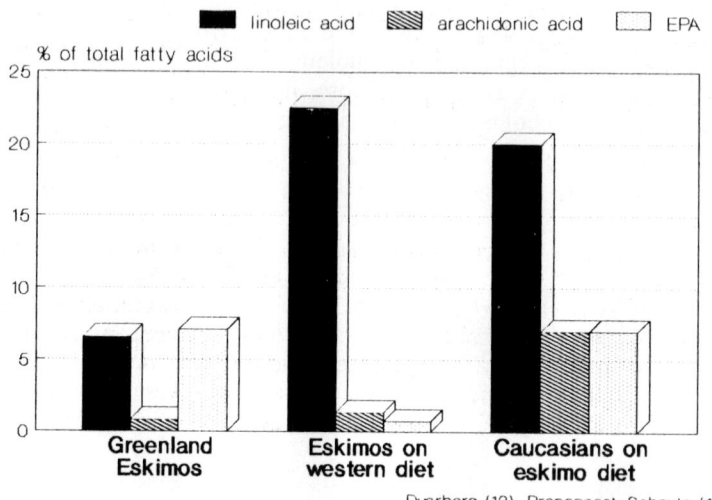

Figure 4. Percentage of linoleic acid, arachidonic acid and eicosapentaenoic acid in plasma phospholipids of Greenland Eskimos on their traditional seafood diet and on western diet and of Caucasians on an Eskimo diet.

Dietary linoleic acid intake and prostaglandin formation

Linoleic acid intake has, according to the above results, two important effects on plasma lipids, i.e. phospholipids, especially lecithin are lowered and the concentration of arachidonic acid in HDL is decreased. Both factors may influence PG-biosynthesis, as lecithin is the pool for precursor substances and arachidonic acid is the main precursor for PG-formation. There is sufficient evidence that PG-biosynthesis is related to the availability of essential fatty acids for the PG synthesizing enzymes [3]. Arachidonic acid infused intraarterially in graded doses provoked a dose-dependent increase of PG-formation in isolated organs of experimental animals [19]. Supplementation of arachidonic acid caused an increased biosynthesis of PG-E_2, probably as a consequence of the enriched precursor pool [20].

Determination of PG-biosynthesis *in vivo* is difficult. Because of the short half-life of eicosanoids, the value of plasma level determinations is limited. Even the measurement of metabolites, which are more stable, reveales considerable cicadiane variations and their production depends on sex hormones and other factors [21, 22]. More reliable for PG-biosynthesis studies are the determinations of stable urinary metabolites in which 80-90% of endogenous PGs are converted. A procedure for the determination of the joint urinary PG-metabolites has been elaborated by Nugteren [23]. Thi method is based on the chemical transformation of C16-metabolites of PG-D, E and F to a stable compound, named tetranorprostanedioic acid.

We have done determinations of urinary PG-metabolites in females on a linoleic acid intake of 0, 10, and 50 g/d [25]. Linoleic acid in cholesterol esters increased with augmented intake from 35% to 63%. At the end of each two weeks period of formula diets PG metabolites transformable to tetranorprostanedioic acid were measured. We found an increase of PG-metabolites with increased linoleic acid intake. According to a linoleic acid intake of 0, 10 or 50 g/d and amount of 123, 175 and 352 µg of urinary PG-metabolites, transformable to tetranorprostanedioic acid, were measured [26]. Nugteren [23] reported a very similar increase of urinary metabolites in rats with augmented linoleic acid intake, indicating a similar stimulation of PG biosynthesis in both species (*figure 5*). Measurements of renal PG in 24-h-urines of these females revealed an icnrease of PG-E_2, while no effect was observed with PG-$F_{2\alpha}$ [27]. PG-E_2 increases renal sodium excretion and renal blood flow. In fact, an increase of renal creatinin and sodium excretion, and of creatinine clearance could be measured with augmented linoleic acid intake in 32 volunteers [27]. Remarkably potassium and water excretion was lowest with a linoleic acid intake between 6 to 8 energy%, which is about the intake with conventional diet.

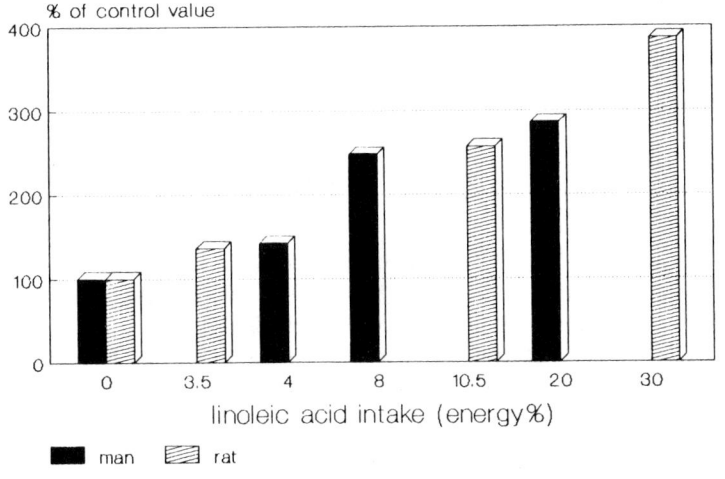

Figure 5. Prostaglandin biosynthesis in man (1) and rats (24) evaluated by the determination of urinary prostaglandin metabolites during diets providing different amounts of linoleic acid.

Essential fatty acids

Nutritional modification of prostaglandin biosynthesis in man

N-3 fatty acids, like alpha-linolenic acid, inhibit PG-formation by competition with n–6 fatty acids for the synthetizing enzymes. This competition has been shown in vitro for the delta-6-desaturase, resulting in a depressed formation of arachidonic acid, which is the main precursor for PG-biosynthesis. As described above, this competition is not very important *in vivo*. Therefore the main effect of n–3 fatty acids occurs at the level of the cyclo-oxygenase, resulting in a depression of PG-biosynthesis from arachidonic acid.

Formation of arachidonic acid from linoleic acid is hardly needed in western communities, because the intake of arachidonic acid, with the meat consumed in western diets, amounts to 100-200 mg/d. The amount of arachidonic acid needed for PG-biosynthesis, about 1 mg/d, is surpassed by far. In one experiment in man, Syberth showed that supplementation of the diet with arachidonic acid resulted in enhanced platelet aggregation, which may lead to arteriosclerosis [20]. Therefore inhibition of cyclo-oxygenase with n–3 fatty acids has been recommlended for the dietary prevention of arteriosclerosis in western communities.

N–3 fatty acids are a poor substrate for the PG-forming enzyme, cyclo-oxygenase, and *in vivo* no appreciable amounts of PG are formed from n–3 fatty acids [28]. If arachidonic acid intake is low, n–3 fatty acids readily diminish PG-formation and platelet aggregation, and increase the bleeding time, was we have shown in volunteers [15]. Collagen-induced platelet aggregation decreased with an alpha-linolenic acid intake of 12 or 16 energy% to 75 or 70% of the control value under conventional diet. An EPA intake of 1.7% resulted in a similar decrease of platelet aggregation

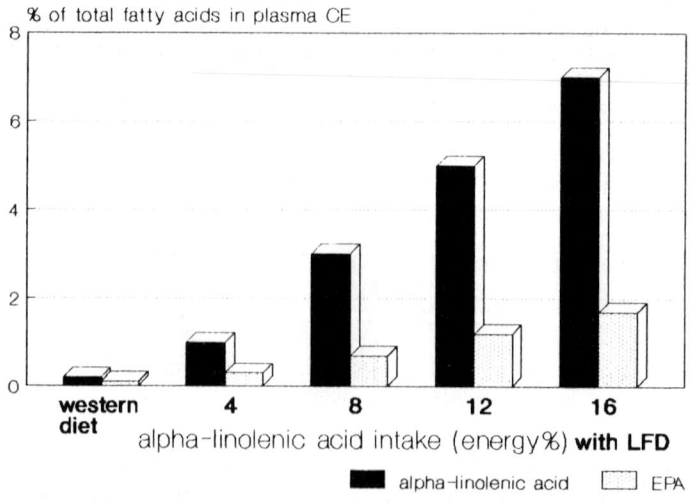

Figure 6. Linolenic and eicosapentaenoic acid (EPA) in plasma cholesterol-esters during LFDs devoid of EPA. Determinations were done in six healthy females (age 23-32 years) at the end of LFDs providing a constant amount of 4 energy% linoleic acid. For periods of two weeks each 4%, 8%, 12% and 16% of alpha-linolenic acid were given.

as an alpha-linolenic acid intake of 16 energy% [15]. Bleeding time increased with an alpha-linolenic acid intake of 12 energy% to 140% of the control value. Again EPA was about tenfold more active in prolonging bleeding time than alpha-linolenic acid.

If the intake of alpha-linolenic acid is increased from 0 to 16 energy%, during a constant linoleic acid supply of 4 energy%, PG-E$_2$ decreases approximately dose-dependent from 254 ± 48 to 35 ± 11 ng/d, while PGF$_{2\alpha}$ only decreases with an alpha-linolenic acid intake of 12 or more energy% [15]. Wether these effects are attributable to alpha-linolenic acid or to endogenous formed EPA is not easily discernible. It should be noted that the effects of alpha-linolenic acid became apparent after the percentage of EPA, which was not provided with the diet, reached 1% of plasma cholesterol fatty acids (*figure 6*). This percentage of EPA also turned out to be effective, if EPA was given with the diet [15].

An adequate PG-formation is warranted in the renal, pulmonary and gastro-intestinal system as well as for hormonal, immunologic and allergic responses of the cell. Because PG serve functions in a multitude of cellular reactions, the inhibition of PG-biosynthesis with n–3 fatty acids may cause side-effects in these systems.

References

1. Adam O. (1985) *Klin. Wochenschr.* 63:731.
2. Alfin-Slater R.B., Aftergood L. (1986) *Physiol. Rev.* 48:758.
3. Dupont J., M.M. Mathias (1969) *Lipids* 4:478.
4. Irvine R.F. (1982) *Biochem. J.* 204:3.
5. Irvine R.F., Dawson R.M.C. (1979) *Biochem. Biophys. Res.* Comm. 91:1399.
6. Adam O., Wolfram G., Zöllner N. (1983) In: Phospholipids and atherosclerosis. P. Avogaro, M. Mancini, F. Ricci, R. Paoletti (eds.), pp 237-260.
7. Lapetina E.G., Billah M.M., Cuatrecasas P. (1978) *Nature* 292:367.
8. Moncada S., Vane J.R. (1978) *Pharmac. Rev.* 30:293.
9. Needleman P., Allery J. (1978) *Clin Immunol.* 26:96.
10. Lewis B. (1980) In: Diet and Drugs in Atherosclerosis. G. Noseda, B. Lewis (eds.), Raven Press, New York, pp 1-8.
11. Brenner R.R., Peluffo R.C. (1966) *Biochim. Biophys. Acta* 176:471.
12. Garcia P.T., Holman R.T. (1965) *J. Am. Oil. Chem. Soc.* 42:1137.
13. Adam O., Wolfram G., Zöllner N. (1986) *J. Lipid Res.* 27:421.
14. Weiner T.W., Sprecher H. (1984) *Biochim. Biophys. Acta* 792:293.
15. Adam O., Wolfram G., Zöllner N. (1986) *Klin. Wochenschr.* 64:274.
16. Dyerberg J., Bang H.O., Hjorne N. (1975) *Am. J. Clin. Nutr.* 28:958.
17. Bronsgeest-Schoute H.C., vanGent C.M., Luten J.B., Ruiter A. (1981) *Am. J. Clin. Nutr.* 34:1752.
18. Dyerberg J., Bang H.O., Stoffersen E., Moncada S., Vane J.R. (1978) *Lancet* i:117.
19. Mentz P., Optiz H., Rettkowski W., Förster W. (1978) *Acta med. germ.* 37:811.
20. Seyberth H.W., Oelz O., Kennedy T. et al. (1975) *Clin. Pharmacol. Ther.* 18:521.
21. Schemmer J.M., Blank M.L., Wykle R.L. (1979) *Prostaglandins* 18:491.
22. Shemesh M., Bensadoun A., Hansel W. (1976) *Proc. Soc. Exp. Biol. Med.* 151:667.

23. Nugteren D.H., vanEvert W.C., Soeting W.J., Spuy J.H. (1980) In: advances in prostaglandin and thromboxane research, Vol 6 and 7:1142, P. Ramwell (ed.). Raven Press, New York.
24. Hornstra G., Christ-Hazelhof E., Haddeman E., tenHoor F., Nugteren D.H. (1981) *Prostaglandins* 21:727.
25. Adam O., Wolfram G., Zöllner N. (1982) *Ann. Nutr. Metab.* 26:315.
26. Zöllner N., Adam O., Wolfram G. (1978) *Res. Exp. Med.* 175:149.
27. Adam O., Wolfram G., Zöllner N. (1984) *Am. J. Clin. Nutr.* 40:415.
28. Mathias M.M., Dumont J. (1985) *LIpids* 20:791.
29. Bierenbaum M.L., Fleischmann A.I., Raichelson R.I., Hayton T., Watson P.B. (1973) *Lancet* I:1404.

Summary

Prostaglandin (PG) biosynthesis depends on the availability of precursor substances and the activity of PG-forming enzymes. Both factors can be influenced by nutritional habits. Dietary linoleic acid is, preferential to other polyunsaturated fatty acids, incorporated into body lipids (1), and gives rise to arachidonic acid, which is the direct PG-precursor. The rate controlling enzyme for the formation of arachidonic acid from linoleic acid (n − 6) in mammalians is the delta-6-desaturase. The activity of this enzyme is regulated *in vivo* by the fatty acid composition of membrane lipids. A high dietary linoleic acid supply decreases the formation of arachidonic acid in man (2). This part of PG-formation is a slow and exact controlled process (3). PG-biosynthesis from membrane-arachidonate occurs within seconds by the activation of the enzyme cyclo-oxigenase upon an appropriate stimulus.

The effect of dietary linoleic acid intake of PG-biosynthesis is difficult to evaluate, because several nutrients are known to affect PG-formation (e.g.vitamin B12, E and C) and because the half-live of PG is so short, that only the determination of metabolites can give an impression of the amount of PG-biosynthesis. We have done determinations of urinary PG-metabolites in females on a linoleic acid intake of 0, 4, and 20 energy% with liquid formula diets. At the end of each two weeks period an amount of 123, 175 and 352 µg of urinary PG-metabolites, were measured (4). In critical ill patients the increase of PG-biosynthesis during parenteral linoleic acid supply was comparable to those results, observed in healthy volunteers. Measurements of renal PG in 24-h-urines revealed an increase of PG-E_2, while no effect was observed with PG-$F_{2\alpha}$. PG-E_2 increases renal sodium excretion and renal blood flow and in fact, an increase of creatinine clearance and of renal sodium excretion could be measured in 32 healthy volunteers during high linoleic acid intake (1). Following high linoleic acid intake an increase of PG-metabolites was found after 4 days. This may be a reflection of the time until linoleic acid has been transformed to arachidonic acid and is available in phospholipids for PG-biosynthesis. A linoleic deficient diet causes a decrease of PG-metabolites within 24 hr. As changes of membrane arachidonate after such a short time cannot be taken into account, other dietary factors may be responsable for the decrease of PG-biosynthesis. Most dietary studies confirm that linoleic acid intake decreases thromboxan A2 formation, resulting in a reduced platelet aggregation. Concerning prostacyclin and leukotrien production the reports in the literature are unaequivocal, depending on the set of experiments.

In summary it can be concluded that oral or parenteral linoleic acid supply is effective in modulating prostaglandin biosynthesis.

Discussion

Dr Bourre: This paper is now open to discussion.

Dr Cunnane: I think that's excellent piece of work, and it's easy to do it in rats but it must be a little bit more difficult to do it with your subjects. My question, if I can be allowed a double barrelled one, is first of all do you have any idea where the prostaglandins are coming from, is it kidney production or is it something released in the circulation which ends up in the urine? And second, can you be certain we have an obvious metabolic link between linoleic acid and prostaglandins, but can you be sure in this setting that linoleic acid is in fact being metabolised for arachidonic acid to make PGs, or is simply stimulating indirectly the release of prostaglandins through some membrane change that's induced without being metabolised 1, 2, 3?

Dr Adam: Two very important questions, I don't know any answers. You know we may assume that native prostaglandins which occur in the urine originate from the kidney, but where from all those other prostaglandins come is just a question which you can't answer. And even the amount is 300 microgram/day, about 300 microgram/day which is a lot. If you look at the PGE metabolites there's only 100 of this, that's about in the range of 20 nanogram/day and so you have to speculate that in this metabolite which we determine there are large amounts of PGD but where from those PGD come, whether from the brain or whether from the intestine or where from ever I can't say but the question which we posed was is by linoleic acid the prostaglandin formation influenced? And that was the point we tried to answer.

Now concerning your second question I can't give any information about this and I showed the data on the decrease of arachidonic acid which would indicate a reduced prostaglandin formation and that's why I believe that actually not the transformation from linoleic acid to arachidonic acid is increased, but membrane function is the real trigger of prostaglandin formation and this would also explain the abrupt effects if you take off the linoleic supply.

Dr Koletzko: You showed these very impressive data on the polytrauma patients with this dramatic decrease of linoleic acid and cholesterol esters. We found through the discussion of this morning. Did you also find a concomitant increase of N–9 eicosatreinoic acid?

Dr Adam: Yes, you can show it.

Prof Navarro: My question concerns also polytraumatic people and about the relationship with Vitamin C in the influence of the biosynthesis of prostaglandins?

Dr Adam: Oh yes, we didn't do any determinations of vitamin C in these patients but it's a very relevant question, but I can't answer it.

Dr Hansen: I would like to pose a question as Chairman. It's very impressive to see the decrease when your giving formula diet without linoleic acid, is that diet anti-inflammatory?

Dr Adam: Actually we are trying now to get any effects of this in this subject but these were healthy volunteers not suffering from any inflammatory disease.

Dr Hansen: I have another one. You showed a picture about increasing the diet from 0 to 20 energy% of linoleic acid measuring the native prostaglandins in urine, and prostaglandin E_2 increased, it doubled. You increase from 0 to 20 that's an enormous increase and you only doubled your prostaglandin production and I agree with you that you can influence prostaglandin formation by its means but also you can also turn that upwards down and say it's not very easy to influence urinary prostaglandins, the native ones, because you have to use enormous amounts of linoleic acid to show the effect.

Dr Adam: That's right, yes, that's a very important point but these studies have been done in totally healthy females and so you could not conclude from this situation to any other illness, something like that.

Dr Huang: It seems you increase from 0 to 20, increase of PGE_2, PGF_1 alpha is not affected would you speculate that maybe PGE_2 in this case can be influenced by dietary, so maybe they are running in a different pool as they produce from the different pool of arachidonic acid for that purpose?

Dr Adam: That's a very important question, some people think that PGF_2 alpha is just a not so effective metabolite of PGE_2, so it's not quite well known what good is PGF_2 alpha for and it's maybe that you are right there two compartments of prostaglandins which are not formed in the same way.

Essential fatty acids and supplemented parenteral nutrition

Table I. Data summary of the 25 general medical surgical (M/S) patients.

Pt. N°.	Age	Sex	Diagnosis	Wt. (kg)	Calculated REE	CHO (kcal)	Fat (kcal)	Prot GM/kg	Total (kcal)	Nitrogen Excretion	Nitrogen Balance	Serum Glucose	Insulin
1	39	F	Bowel obstruction	43	1780	1270	550	1.5	1820	4.0	(+) 6.6	85	0
2	73	M	Pneumonia	54	1840	680	1100	1.0	1780	8.0	(−) 4.4	100	0
3	31	M	Candida sepsis (AIDS)	64	2330	1430	1000	1.9	2430	14.6	(+) 3.0	118	0
4	80	F	Pancreatic carcinoma	40	1380	680	550	.8	1230	--	--	100	0
5	23	M	Ulcerative colitis	54	2100	1530	550	1.6	2080	7.0	(+) 3.6	139	0
6	60	F	Pancreatic abscess	63	1680	1020	550	1.3	1570	4.6	(+) 5.0	260	(+)
7	47	M	Pancreatitis	49	1840	760	1000	1.8	1760	7.0	(+) 1.0	153	0
8	20	M	Ruptured spleen	75	2770	1700	1000	1.1	2700	--	--	114	0
9	39	F	Pancreatic carcinoma	47	1800	850	1000	1.5	1850	10.0	(−) 3.0	106	0
10	33	F	Alcoholic cirrhosis	45	1800	680	1000	1.9	1680	5.4	(+) 3.6	169	(+)
11	74	M	Esophageal carcinoma	67	1830	680	1100	.8	1780	8.0	(−) 4.0	220	0
12	31	M	Crohn's disease	55	2050	1530	550	1.2	2080	5.6	(+) 1.4	96	0
13	62	M	Lymphoma	65	2130	1190	550	1.6	1740	6.8	(+) 5.3	129	0
14	67	M	Aspiration pneumonia	60	1950	680	1100	.9	1780	4.6	--	117	0
15	62	M	UGI bleed	117	3150	950	1000	1.2	1950	7.4	(+) 7.0	113	0
16	45	F	Esophageal stricture	91	2470	850	1000	1.3	1850	7.5	(+) 8.5	107	0
17	22	F	Ulcerative colitis	46	1250	1020	550	1.7	1570	5.5	(+) 2.5	117	0
18	32	M	Hodgin's lymphoma	78	2700	710	1000	.9	1710	28.3	(−) 17.3	153	0
19	25	M	(AIDS) encephalitis	61	2370	1020	1100	1.3	2120	12.0	--	103	0
20	74	M	Pneumonia	60	1870	680	1100	.9	1780	--	--	134	0
21	73	F	Colon carcinoma	83	1900	950	1000	1.3	1950	--	--	110	0
22	40	M	Gunshot wounds	77	2640	1190	1000	1.3	2190	10.9	(+) 1.1	149	0
23	43	M	Atypical sprue	47	1770	714	1000	1.5	1710	4.0	(+) 3.4	142	0
24	97	F	Bowel obstruction	45	1420	680	550	1.2	1230	--	--	93	0
25	87	F	Dysphagia	62	1620	1040	550	.6	1590	10.8	(−) 8.8	104	0

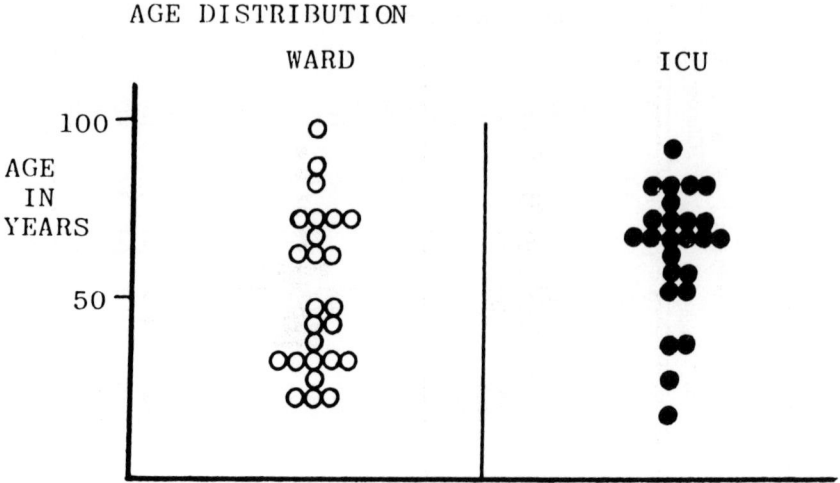

Figure 1. Age distribution of the two patient groups. (Each circle represents one patient).

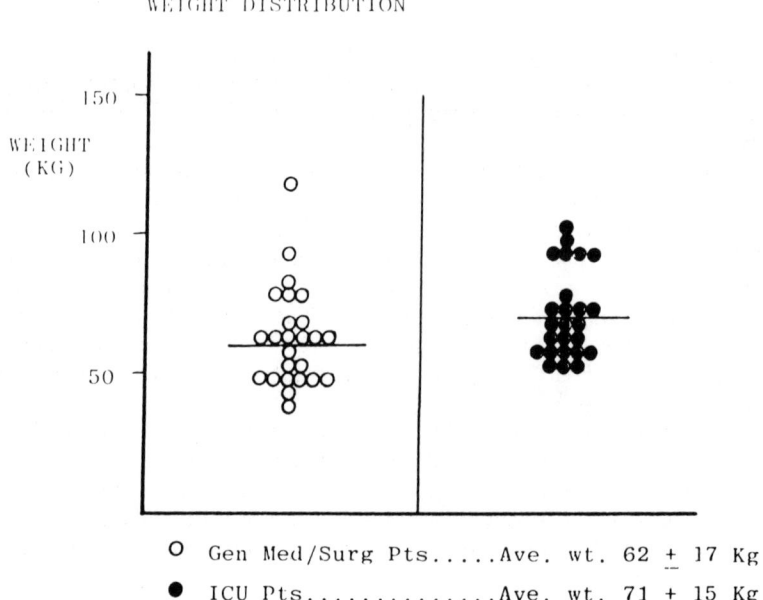

Figure 2. Weight distribution of the two patient groups (Each circle represents one patient).

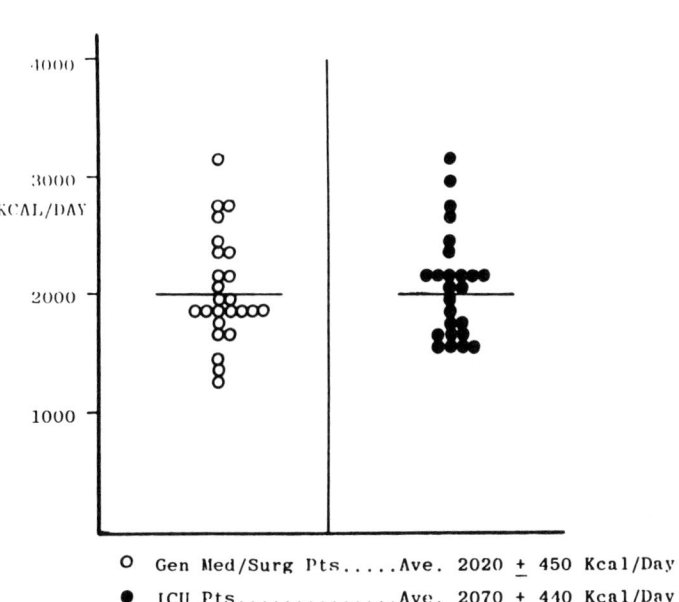

Figure 3. Distribution of the calculated resting energy expenditure for the two patient groups. (Each circle represents one patient).

The initial nutritional support prescription for the two groups recommended on average slightly more than 1800 kilocalories/day (*figure 4*). Approximately 50% of these calories were supplied as carbohydrate (*figure 5*) and 50% as fat (*figure 6*).

The protein intake for the M/S ward patients averaged 1.28 ± 0.35 gm/kg and 1.26 ± 0.41 gm/kg for the ICU patients. This level of intake had 14 of the 21 ICu patients for whom balance data was available in zero or positive nitrogen balance within three to seven days of initiation of nutritional support (*figure 7*). Similarly 15 of the 20 M/S ward patients with balance data available were in zero to positive nitrogen balance within seven days of initiation of therapy (*figure 7*). Nitrogen excretion for the two groups is shown in *figure 8*. The M/S patients averaged excretion of 8.60 <145 5.3 gms/day compared to the 12.68 ± 7.85 gms/day excreted by the ICU patients. This would correspond to the greater severity of illness and stress seen in the ICU patients.

The relationship between kilocalorie intake and nitrogen excretion is shown in *figure 9*. There was no correlation shown between kilocalorie intake and nitrogen excretion. Exogenous insulin was required for control of serum glucose in 3 (12%) of the ICU patients all of whom were insulin requiring diabetics prior to this acute hospitalization (*Table II*). Similarly the two M/S patients who required insulin were also diabetic (*Table I*).

Table II. Data summary of the 25 intensive care (ICU) patients.

Pt. N°.	Age	Sex	Diagnosis	Wt. (kg)	Calculated REE	Measured REE	RQ	CHO (kcal)	Fat (kcal)	Prot GM/kg	Total (kcal)	Nitrogen Excretion	Balance	Glucose	Insulin
1	72	M	Colon perforation	65	2130	1900	.78	630	800	1.4	1430	10.0	(+) 1.5	167	0
2	55	M	Aortic aneurysm	74	2470	2300	1.00	1190	1000	2.3	2190	17.8	(−) 4.1	174	0
3	84	F	Bowel infarction	90	2100	--	--	710	1000	1.2	1710	6.6	(+) 5.3	93	0
4	15	F	Appendiceal abscess	56	2190	--	--	1530	2000	2.0	3530	22.7	(+) 2.0	102	0
5	80	F	Diverticulitis	54	1540	--	--	680	1000	.9	1680	--	--	120	0
6	50	M	Closed head injury	54	1870	--	--	760	1000	1.5	1760	15.4	(−) 6.1	149	0
7	74	F	Gastric carcinoma	57	1690	--	--	680	500	.9	1180	6.3	(−) 2.3	121	0
8	58	M	Cardiac transplant	98	2917	--	--	1600	1000	1.0	2600	--	--	211	(+)
9	65	M	Pancreatic carcinoma	93	2660	--	--	1420	1000	1.3	2420	12.5	(+) 2.5	185	(+)
10	64	F	Breast carcinoma	79	2090	2000	.90	950	1000	.3	1950	16.8	(−) 4.0	203	0
11	67	F	Colovesicle fistula	50	1560	--	--	680	1000	1.0	1680	--	--	233	0
12	65	F	Mistral insufficiency	60	1770	1200	.70	710	1000	1.0	1710	--	--	220	0
13	69	M	Pyelonephritis	104	2790	--	--	950	1000	1.3	1950	6.5	(+) 2.3	107	0
14	74	F	Pancreatitis	91	2170	2400	.90	2140	(MWF)	2.0	2140	14.9	(+) 5.6	157	0
15	26	M	Quadriplegia	91	3160	1900	.90	1190	1000	1.5	2190	41.0	(−) 18.0	127	0
16	65	M	Bowel obstruction	72	2160	1900	.76	850	550	1.6	1400	13.3	(+) 2.7	104	0
17	92	F	Bowel obstruction	58	1500	1450	.78	890	550	1.3	1440	12.4	(+) 3.2	198	0
18	71	F	Cholecystitis	59	1680	1730	.72	590	1000	1.0	1590	4.0	(+) 1.5	242	0
19	51	M	Legionaires disease	72	2340	--	--	1070	1000	1.2	2070	13.9	(−) 1.3	253	(+)
20	39	F	Cholecystitis	70	2140	--	--	1360	550	1.2	1910	13.3	(−) 3.7	170	0
21	77	M	Aortic dissection	66	1930	--	--	890	1000	1.0	1890	8.4	(+) 2.9	181	0
22	68	F	Bowel obstruction	68	1530	--	--	590	550	1.0	1140	5.0	(−) 2.2	103	0
23	81	F	Colon carcinoma	60	1660	--	--	850	1000	.8	1850	6.7	(+) 5.7	117	0
24	83	F	Pulmonary embolus	64	1780	--	--	710	1000	1.4	1710	9.9	--	215	0
25	36	F	Closed head injury	59	2010	--	--	950	1000	1.4	1950	8.9	(+) 0.7	125	0

Essential fatty acids and supplemented parenteral nutrition

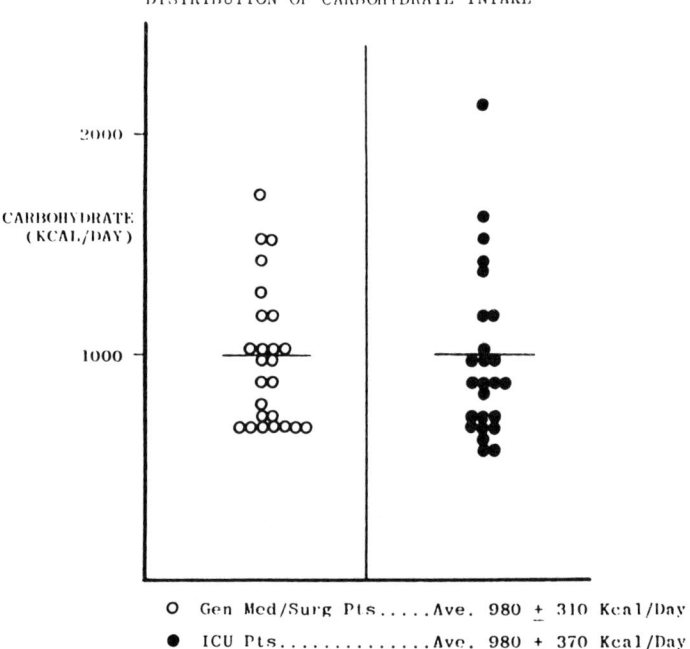

Figure 4. Distribution of the carbohydrate intake for the two patient groups (Each circle represents one patient).

Discussion

Initially three polyunsaturated fatty acids were considered essential for the prevention of EFAD. These were: arachidonic acid (20:4w6), linoleic acid (18:2w6) and linolenic acid (18:3w3). Arachidonic acid ceased to be regarded as an essential dietary component after Steinberg *et al.* in 1956 demonstrated that arachidonic acid could be synthesized *in vivo* from linoleic acid [10].

Linoleic acid continues to be accepted as an essential nutrient for two reasons: a) it cannot be synthesized *in vivo* and b) it has a defined metabolic significance. Administration of only 1 to 2% of dietary calories in the form of linoleic acid will support normal growth and development and prevent the clinical appearance of EFAD [11, 12]. In the weanling rat, growth can be related logarithmically to the intake of linoleic acid (12-13). In the deficient animal, linoleic acid will reverse all of the known clinical manifestations of EFAD [11, 13].

The position of linolenic acid as a essential nutrient is controversial. It, like linoleic acid, cannot be synthesized *in vivo*, but the metabolic significance of linolenic acid is not clear. Administration of linolenic acid will reverse some, but not all of the manifestations of EFAD. For example, the reproductive failure associated with EFAD is not reversed by linolenate administration, but is with linolate

Essential fatty acids

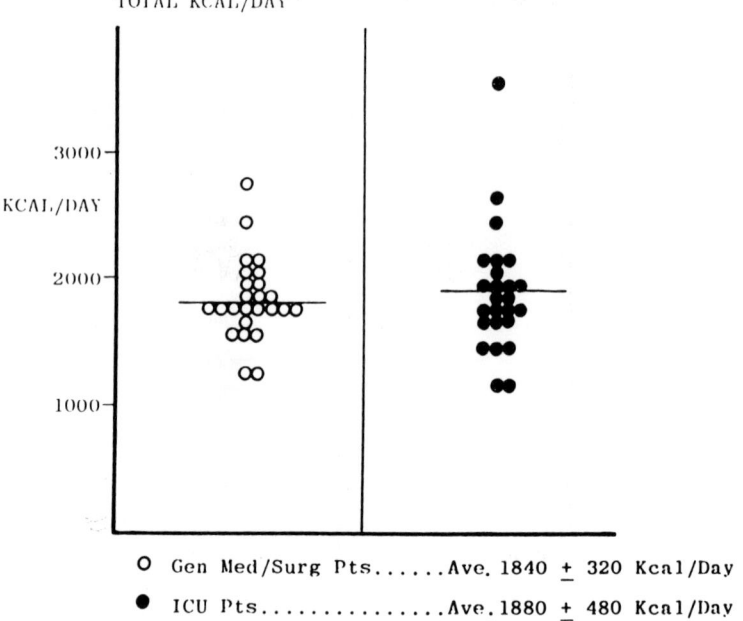

Figure 5. Distribution of the total kilocalorie (kcal) per day intake for the two groups of patients. (Each circle represents one patient).

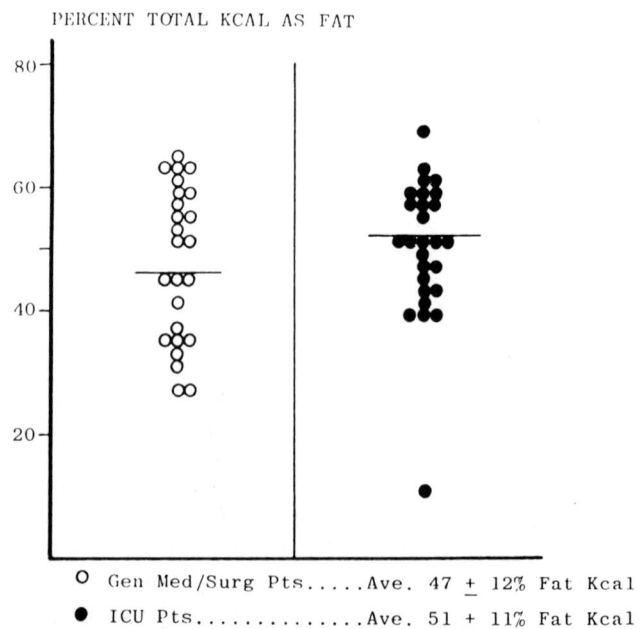

Figure 6 Display of percent of total kilocalories per day administered as intravenous fat emulsion. (Each circle represents one patient).

Essential fatty acids and supplemented parenteral nutrition

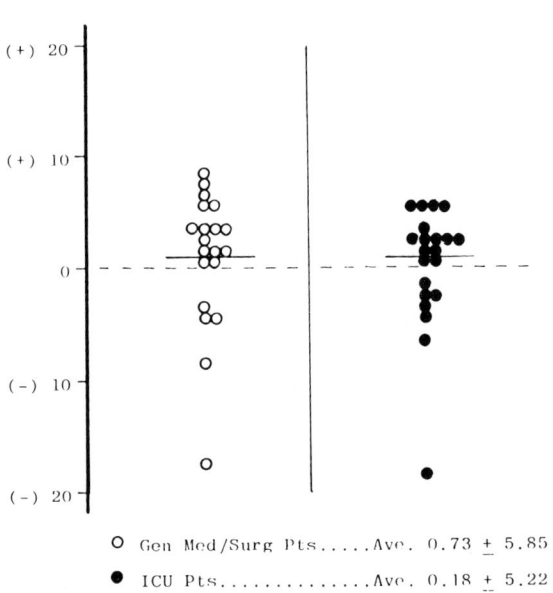

Figure 7. Display of the nitrogen balance data for the two groups of patients. (Each circle represents one patient).

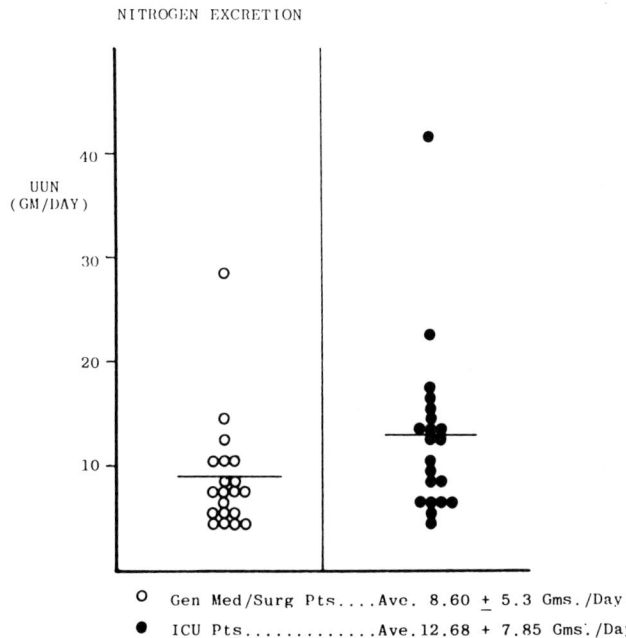

Figure 8. Display of nitrogen excretion for the two groups of patients. (Each circle represents one patient).

Essential fatty acids

[11, 13]. Linolenic acid does not support growth as effectively as linoleic acid, nor is linolenic acid as effective as linoleic acid in correcting the abnormal skin permeability seen with EFAD [11, 13]. In short, linolenic acid has not been defined as essential in terms of classical EFAD. Some investigators have speculated, however, that linolenic acid may be essential in determining the polyunsaturated acid composition and function of some specialized body tissues [14, 17].

Attempts to define an essential role for linolenic acid have focused on the structure and function of tissues with a high content of w3. The metabolites of linolenic acid are found as structural components of brain and retinal tissue phospholipids and precursors of the triene prostaglandins [17]. Docosahexaenoic acid (22:6w3) is a component of human cerebral cortex, retina and muscle [18]. Eicosapentanoic (20:5w3) is the immediate precursor of the triene prostaglandins including prostaglandin E_3, thromboxane A_3 and prostacyclin I_3B Both docosahexaenoic acid and eicosapentanoic acid can be synthesized to some extent *in vivo* in man and other species [17, 19]. Only a small amount of exogenously administered linolenic is metabolized to these two acids [17, 19, 20]. In particular, eicosapentanoic acid associated with decreased atherosclerosis and prolonged bleeding times in some populations is ingested for the most part performed in dietary oils [21, 23].

Despite knowledge of the end-products of linolenic acid metabolism, no convincing and reproducible linolenic acid deficienty has yet been demonstrated [10, 13]. A wealth of data, however, indicates that w3 fatty acids and their metabolites have

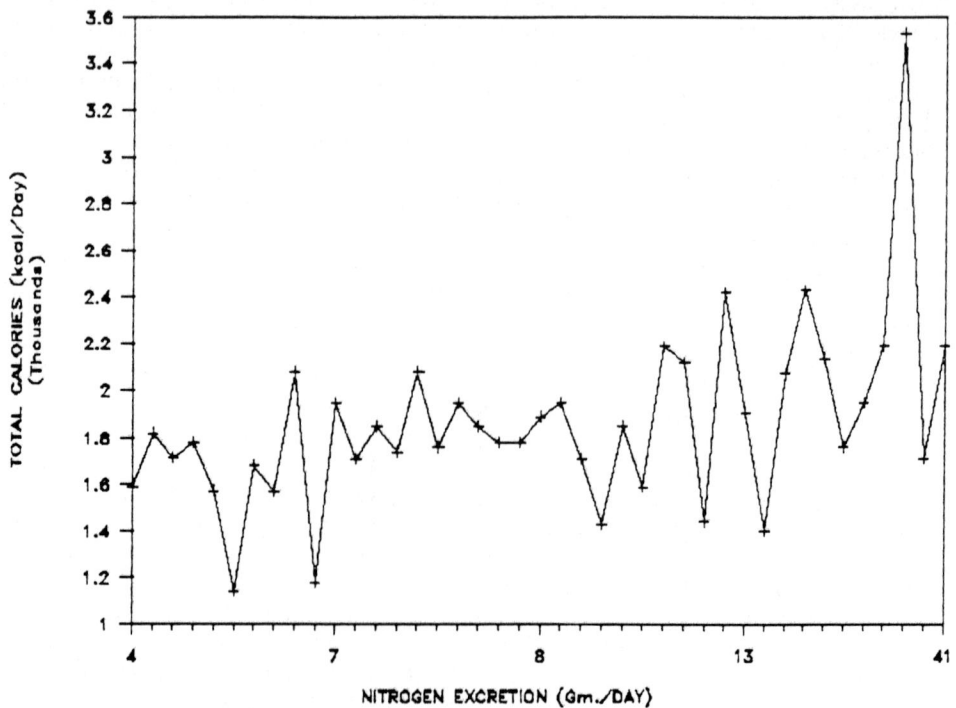

Figure 9. Graphic plot of nitrogen excretion versus total calories for the two groups of patients.

competitive and inhibitory effects on the metabolism of the linoleic (w6) fatty acids [10, 13]. Only 0.1% of calories as linolenic acid are required to induce a 50% inhibition of the metabolic conversion of linoleic acid to 22:5w6 [11]. An absolute or relative excess of linolenic acid intake results in abnormal fatty acid metabolite profiles and membrane structure [10, 12]. Most of the abnormalities following excess linolenic acid intake can be ascribed to the preferential incorporation of w3 fatty acids into membrane phospholipids [23, 24]. Other mechanisms, such as vitamin E deficiency and prostaglandin imbalance also appear to be involved but their importance is incompletely defined [25].

Although the nutritional advantages and safe administration of intravenous lipid emulsions in humans were reported as early as 1935, it was not until 1947 that Hansen suggested an exogenous source of the polyunsaturated fatty acids of the w6 family was essential in humans [26]. In the late 1950's, Lipomul I.V., composed of 15% cottonseed oil and Pluronic-F 68 as the emulsifying agent, was marketed as a source of parenteral calories [27]. While early reports of increased weight gain and nitrogen retention were encouraging, further investigation yielded adverse reactions following multiple infusions of Lipomul which included abnormal liver function tests, hepatomegaly, splenomegaly, accumulation of "sudanophilic" material in the liver, anorexia, fever and thrombocytopenia [28, 31]. Catastrophes following Lipomul infusion were termed the "fat overload syndrome" and led to abandonment of fat emulsions for parenteral nutrition in the United States [32]. In the late 1960's a new method for the administration of hyperosmolar solutions of glucose, protein hydrolysates, vitamins and electrolytes via the subclavian vein brought prolonged parenteral nutrition to hospitalized patients and a consequent clinical appreciation of EFAD [1, 3, 33, 34]. Research is still needed to determine optimal amounts of essential fatty acids required in hospitalized patients. Most studies indicate that 4% of the total non-protein caloric intake of linoleic acid will effectively reverse clinical and biochemical signs of EFAD and prevent their occurrence [1, 3].

Although the primary use of fat emulsions has been to prevent EFAD, attention in the last few years has been given to the use of fat emulsions as a substantial source of calories in the hospitalized patient. In the clinical series of patients reported here, assessing the "optimal" infusion of fat emulsion on clinical grounds ordinarily led to providing 40 – 60% of calories as lipid. This approach was associated with a positive nitrogen balance within seven days of therapy in 75% of our general medical/surgical ward patients and 66% of our intensive care unit patients. This regimen has decreased the insulin required to control hyperglycemia particularly in the stressed critically ill intensive care unit patient. Benefits in terms of decreased respirator dependence because of reduced carbon dioxide production or more efficient calorie utilization are less easily defined. It should be emphasized that the data presented here are the response to the initial nutritional perscription. After evaluation of glucose tolerance, respiratory quotient, energy expenditure, nitrogen balance and serum triglycerides, as well as other clinical parameters, the nutrition regimen should be modified in an attempt to optimize the clinical response.

Although it seems clear that the utility of parenteral fat emulsions is firmly established both to prevent EFAD and as a primary calorie source much work needs to be done to define "what is essential and optimal" for specific clinical objectives. For example, in the severely stressed patient can fat infusion serve to conserve protein [35, 37]? In this clinical series and in our previous work with head-injured patients no correlation could be found between non-protein calorie administration and protein catabolism [38, 39]. This data suggests that protein conservation does not occur in the severely stressed patient or that the appropriate calorie source has not been found. Could alternative fat emulsions perhaps composed of medium chain triglycerides play a role in protein conservation? It is known that fatty acids play a role in the prostaglandin system. Recently, Trocki *et al.* have suggested that fatty acids impact on immunity in the burned animal [40]. Can manipulation of the fatty acid substrate used for nutritional support be effective in helping the compromised patient deal with a septic challenge? Bahrami et al have suggested that intravenous fat infusions may favorably influence lung surfactant [8]. Can a fat emulsion be designed that will provide a means of treating or at least improving the outcome of adult respiratory distress syndrome? These are just a few examples of the types of clinical problems that can be considered from the perspective of what is "essential and optimal" in the use and study of fat emulsions in human nutrition.

References

1. O. Neill J.A., Caldwell M.D., Meng H.C. (1977) Essential fatty acid deficiency in surgical patients. Ann. Surg. 185:535.
2. Bivins B.A., Rapp R.P., Record K.E. et al (1980) Parenteral safflower oil emulsion (Liposyn 10%): Safety and effectiveness in treating or preventing essential fatty acid deficiency in surgical patients. Ann. Surg. 191:307.
3. Goodgame J.T., Lowry S.F., Brennan M.F. (1978) Esential fatty acid deficiency in total parenteral nutrition: Time course of development and suggestions for therapy. *Surgery* 84:271.
4. Skolnik P., Eaglstein W.H., Ziloh V.A. (1977) Human essential fatty acid deficiency. *Arch. Dermatol.* 113:939.
5. Richardson T.J., Sgoutas D. (1975) Essential fatty acid deficiency in four adult patients during total parenteral nutrition. Am. J. Clin. Nutr. 28:258.
6. Twyman D.L., Rapp R.P., Bivins B.A. (1982) Fat emulsions as a calorie source int otal parenteral nutrition: A review of metabolism in fasted, traumatized, septic and normal man. (Part I) Am. J. Iv Ther Clin Nutr 9:11.
7. Twyman D.L., Rapp R.P., Bivins B.A. (1982) Fat emulsions as a calorie source in total parenteral nutrition: A review of metabolism in fasted, traumatized, septic and normal man. (Part II) Am. J. Iv. Ther. Clin. Nutr. 9:9.
8. Bahrami S., Strohmaier W., Redl H., Schlag G. (1987) Mechanical properties of the lungs of posttraumatic rats are improved by including fat in total parenteral nutrition. *J. Parent. Ent. Nutr.* 11:560.
9. Bivins B.A., Bell R.M., Rapp R.P. Griffen W.O. (1983) Linoleic acid vesus linolenic acid: What is essential? J. Parent. Ent. Nutr. 7:473.
10. Steinberg K.G., Seston W.H., Howton D.R. et al (1956) Metabolism of essential fatty acids: IV. Incorporation of linoleate into arachidonic acid. J. Biol. Chem. 220:257.
11. Holman R.T. (1964) Nutritional and metabolic interrelationships between fatty acids. *Proc. Fed. Am. Soc. Exp. Biol.* 23:1062.
12. Holman R.T. (1970) Essential fatty acid deficiency. Prog; Chem. Fats Lipids 9:275.
13. Houtomuller U.M.T. (1975) Specific biological effects of polyunsaturated fatty acids. In: *The role of fats in human nutrition.* Vergroessen A.J. (ed). Academic Press, London, pp. 331.

14. Fiennes R.N.T.-W., Sinclair A.J., Crawford M.A. (1973) essential fatty acid studies in primates: Linolenic acid requirements of capuchins. *J. Med. Prim.* 2:155.
15. Benolken R.M., Anderson R.E., Wheeler T.G. (1973) Membrane fatty acids associated with the electrical response in visual excitation. *Science* 18:1253.
16. Crawford M.A., Hassam A.G., Rivers J.P.W. (1978) Essential fatty acid requirements infancy. *Am. J. Clin. Nutr.* 31:2181.
17. Tinoco J., Babcock R., Hincenbergs I. et al. (1979) Linolenic acid deficiency. *Lipids* 14:166.
18. Alexander M.A.J. (1980) Use of lipid. In: *Nutrition in clinical surgery*, Deitel M. (ed), Williams and Wilkins, Baltimore, pp. 83.
19. Gryglewski R.J., Salmon J.A., Ubatuba F.B. et al. (1979) Effects of all cis-5, 8, 11, 14, 17 eicosapentanoic acid and PGH_3 on platelet aggregation. *Prostaglandins* 18:453.
20. Dyerberg J., Bang H.O., Aagaard O. (1980) Alpha-Linolenic acid and eicosapentanoic acid. *Lancet* 1:199.
21. Dyerberg J., Baug H.O., Hjrne N. (1975) Fatty acid composition of the plasma lipid in Greenland Eskimos. *Am. J. Clin. Nutr.* 28:958.
22. Von Lossonczy T.O., Ruiter A., Brongeest-Schoute H.C. et al. (1978) The effect of a fish diet on serum lipids in healthy human subjects. *Am. J. Clin. Nutr.* 31:1340.
23. Saunders T.A.B., Ellis F.R., Dickerson J.W.T. (1978) Studies of vegans: The fatty acid composition of plasma choline phosphoglycerides, erythrocytes, adipose tissue, and breast milk, and some indicators of susceptibility to ischemic heart disease in vegans and omnivore controls. *Am. J. Clin. Nutr.* 31:805.
24. Bryant P.J., Clawson K.D., Bivins B.A. et al. (1982) Changes in red cell membrane fatty acids in patients receiving total parenteral nutrition supplemented with a safflower oil emulsion. *J. Parent Ent. Nutr.* 6:200.
25. Gudbjarnson S., Hallgrimsson J. (1974) The role of myocardial membrane lipids in the development of cardiac necrosis. In *Proceedings of the international study group for research cardiac metabolism*. Kolbel F (ed), Academic Press, London, pp. 17.
26. Hansen A.E., Knott E.M., Shaperman E., Mc Quarre I. (1947) Eczema and essential fatty acids. *Am. J. Dis. Child.* 73:1.
27. Bozian R.C., Davidson N.W., Stutman L.J., Wilkinson C.F. (1957) Observations on the use of intravenous fat emulsions in man. *Metab. Clin. Exp.* 6:703.
28. Artz C.P., Williams T.K. (1957) The protein-sparing effect of intravenous fat emulsion. *Metab. Clin. Exp.* 6:682.
29. Abbott W.E. (1957) Effect of intravenously administered fat on body weight and nitrogen balance in surgical patients. *Metab. Clin. Exp.* 6:703.
30. Watkin D.M. (1957) Clinical, chemical, hematologic, and anatomic changes accompanying repeated intravenous administration of fat emulsion to man. *Metab. Clin. Exp.* 6:785.
31. Levenson S.M., Upjohn H.L., Sheehy T.W. (1957) Two severe reactions following the long-term infusion of large amounts of intravenous fat emulsion. *Metab. Clin. Exp.* 6:807.
32. Belin R.P., Bivins B.A., Jona J.Z., Young V.L. (1976) Fat overload with a 10% soybean oil emulsion. *Arch. Surg.* 111:1391.
33. Caldwell M.D., Jonsson H.T., Otherson H.B. (1957) Essential fatty acid deficiency in an infant receiving prolonged parenteral alimentation. *J. Pediat.* 81:894.
34. Collins F.D., Sinclair A.J., Royle J.P. et al. (1971) Plasma lipids in human linoleic acid deficiency, *Nutr. Metab.* 13:150.
35. Rakinic J., Takimoto G., Barrett J.A. et al. (1987) Adipose tissue response to insulin following injury. *J. Parent. Ent. Nutr.* 11:513.
36. Gilder H. (1986) Parenteral nourishment of patients undergoing surgical or traumatic stress. *J. Parent. Ent. Nutr.* 10:88.
37. Long C.L. (1987) Fuel preferences int he septic patient: glucose or lipid? *J. Parent Ent. Nutr.* 11:333.

38. Twyman D.L., Bivins B.A. (1986) Nutritional support of the brain injured patient: Five years of clinical study in perspective. *Henry Ford Hosp. Med. J.* 34:41.
39. Bivins B.A., Twyman D.L., Young A.B. (1986) Failure of non-protein calories to mediate protein conservation in brain-injured patients. *J. Trauma* 26:980.
40. Trocki O., Heyd T.J., Waymack J.P., Alexander J.W. (1987) Effects of fish oil on postburn metabolism and immunity. *J. Parent. Ent. Nutr.* 11:521.

Summary

The general availability of safe effective intravenous fat emulsions has changed the clinical question from "what is essential" to the question of "what is optimal". Our patients routinely receive 500 ml of a 10% fat emulsion daily as part of their initial total parenteral nutrition (TPN) regimen. Alterations in the fat composition of this initial regimen are based on: (1) glucose tolerance, (2) respiratory quotient and (3) measured energy expenditure.

We have compared the clinical course of 25 intensive care patients and 25 general medical/surgical ward patients with respect to requirements for intravenous fat emulsion. Parameters monitored included: (1) serum glucose, (2) insulin requirements, (3) nitrogen balance, (4) respiratory quotient and (5) measured energy expenditure. In general terms our severely stressed intensive care patients were more likely to be glucose intolerant and to require a higher proportion of infused calories as fat. As we have previously reported nitrogen excretion did not seem to correlate with calorie infusion, but did correlate with nitrogen infusion. Assessing the "optimal" infusion of fat emulsion on clinical grounds ordinarily leads to providing 40-60% of calories as lipid. This approach has decreased the insulin required to control hyperglycemia particularly in the critically ill. Benefits in terms of decreased respirator dependence and more efficient calorie utilization are less easily defined. Work needs to be done to define "what is essential and optimal" in terms of fat emulsion formulation to achieve specific clinical responses.

Discussion

Dr Friedman: We have had also the opportunity to correlate the infusion of parenteral fat emulsions with pulmonary pressure. What do you think about correlation between protein intake and pulmonary hypertension.

Dr Bivins: We have looked at that specifically in our unit; part of the problem is that our practice is to give relatively high protein intakes, particularly to the order of 1.5 to 2.5 per kilo, and have not seen an increase of pulmonary pressure or pulmonary vascular resistance again. That problem is much more commonly a problem in the paediatric age group than it is in the adults. We have also seen a change in pulmonary diffusion capacity with high fat infusions.

Dr Friedman: Pulmonary diffusion is controversial. The other comment I have is that we have studied the pulmonary surfactant with babies with EFA deficiency and did in fact demonstrate at least by chemically abnormal surfactant.

Dr Bjerve (Trondheim): You stated something like that the question of essentiality of fatty acids were not the important issue any longer and you said something to the effect that we are now supplementing essential fat with a great deal of yeast and a great deal of regularity. And that is correct for the type of patients you described, but there are I think several types of patient populations where that is not correct. The out patient, where the cystic fibrosis feeded as an out patient, at least in Norway, that's not correct. The pre-term infants at least in Norway that's not correct. The very old patient living in homes for the elderly that's certainly not correct. So I think although your statement is correct for a lot of the patients that are sick enough to get hospitalized or treated in a 1000 bed hospital. It's not correct al least in Norway for the small units of 10, 15, 20 beds of people that's only old or they are not able to take care of themselves. Then your statement is not correct and I think your final statement about trying to find the optimal way of supplying EFA also for those will apply. That is my feeling and I think we shall not forget those groups of patients as well.

Dr Bivins: I agree with you totally and I emphasize that I was talking about the adult hospitalized patient, the groups that you specified the elderly, the chronically protein calorie malnourished populations in general, are not because a technology is not there to provide them with an adequate nutrition substrate it's because of their other problems preventing them from receiving it. The neonate, the terribly ill paedriatic patient represents a different metabolic problem. This is the general ward hospitalized patient and this the group where I think that we're on the verge of some very exciting discoveries of using nutritional substrates as pharmocologic tools rather than as pure dietary supplements and I think we have moved through three phases really, we're now into the third phase and probably the most exciting phase. The first was repletion truly scurvy if you will, the second was in by passing the gastro-intestinal track by chemically defined diets and by parenteral nutrition and serving to more completely nourish the patient and now we're at a point where we can begin to manipulate the hormonal, enzymatic and target organ response but very specific substrate manipulations in terms of what we administer these patients and it's going to be an extremely complex, difficult period with very very high rewards, the zinc data that we were presented early is a relatively simplistic presentation of something that varies enormously whether the patient is acute or chronic in terms of protein calorie malnutrition as zinc redistributes in the acute phase or is zinc deficient in the chronic phase so the complexity of how we look at these issues as we begin therapeutic interventions apart from just nutrition would be very very exciting.

Dr Adam: You indicated that alpha-linolenic acid is a strong inhibitor of prostaglandin formation and in our studies with alpha-linolenic acid this was not the case in humans. We needed 16 energy % of alpha-linolenic acid in the diet to inhibit prostaglandin formation in terms of platelet diminuation of platelet aggregation or excretion of PGE_2 in 24h urine or excretion of the metabolite or joint matabolite which I presented. So I would ask you whether this is a statement of yourself or other authors.

Dr Bivins: That's from Dr Alexander's laboratory in Cincinatti. You were using healthy volunteers, he was using a rat with a 50% 30° mark and the data made that translate directly. Or he was also the diet he was administering was very low in linoleic acid and very high in linolenic acid so it may have to do with the absolute ratio rather than the calorie per cent.

9

Metabolic utilization of linoleic acid from fat emulsion during total parenteral nutrition in infants. Fatty acids composition of lipid tissues and prostaglandin synthesis

Z. FRIEDMAN

Neonatalogy, Department of Pediatrics, Baylor College of Medicine, 1200 Moursund Ave, Houston, Texas, 77030 USA

Since some plasma fatty acids reflect tissue fatty acids, we wanted to study it in the newborn and we measured the per cent fatty acid composition of multiple tissues in fœtuses and in newborns. This study basically demonstrates for example in renal tissue (*figure 1*) three important points, one that the arachidonic acid is significantly increased also linoleic acid throughout this period of gestation from 16-44 weeks; two, that if we want to look at the per cent fatty acid composition of these two fatty acids, there is really very little change or no change along this period of gestation; and three in fact the levels of linoleic and arachidonic acids of plasma phospholipids of mothers were not similar to that found in cord plasma phospholipids (*figure 2*). So we postulated that the low tissue level of linoleic acid contribute to low level of linoleic acid in the plasma, in the fœtal plasma and thus increased the gradient concentration between the maternal to the fœtal circulation which could enhance the transfer of this fatty acid across the placenta. What happened with the arachidonic acid and docosahexaenoic acid, we postulated two mechanisms or combinations of them. One is that it could be preferential transfer of these fatty acids across the placenta, and two they could represent increased synthetic activity in the fœtus or the placenta. We measured the specific enzyme activity involved in fatty acid synthesis delta 9 desaturase, in the liver and placenta tissues that were obtained at 8, 16, 18, 20 and 26 weeks of gestation. We found enzymatic activities of these enzymes in the liver and the placenta and in the liver significantly higher than that of the placenta. We don't have any results yet on delta 5 or delta 6 desaturase. Since the EFAs incorporated into phospholipids give basically two important func-

Essential fatty acids

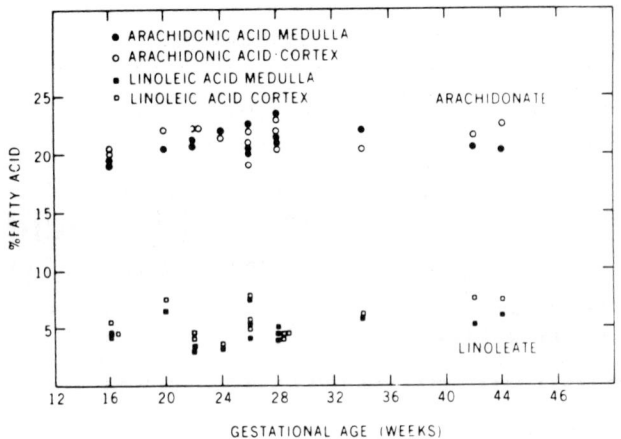

Figure 1. Percent fatty acid composition of renal phospholipids in neonates at various gestional ages. No changes are seen between levels of linoelate and arachidonate in renal tissue beyond 16 weeks of gestation.

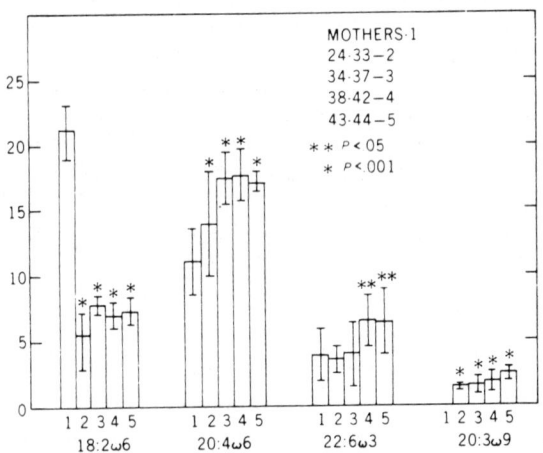

Figure 2. Percent fatty acid composition of plasma phospholipids of mothers and their infants born at varying gestational ages. Note that relative percent of linoleic acid (18:2 ω 6) is lower in cord plasma phospholipids than in maternal plasma; however, levels of arachidonate (20:4 ω 6), docosahexaenoic acid (22:6 ω 3), and Δ-5,8,11-eicosatrienoic acid (20:3 ω 9) are higher in cors plasma than maternal plasma. Relative percent of latter acids increased with advancing gestational age. Ranges in key refer to gestational ages expressed in weeks.

tions, one is that they are stated as a structural function of some membranes and enzymes and the other function is that they are precursor for the eicosanoids. We have done several studies to study the ontology of biosynthetic and degradating enzymes for prostaglandin systems in fœtuses and newborns (*Table I*). We measured these several tissues and I'll just present for you very briefly the results that were

Table I. Clinical data for study groups

Subjects	Sex M	Sex F	Gestational age (wks)	Birth weight (g)	Diagnosis	Vascular tissue studied
1	1		16	225	Abortus	DA, PA, AO
2		1	18	280	Abortus	DA, PA, AO
3	1		26	840	HMD, ICH	DA, PA, AO
4	1		35	1 980	HMD	DA, PA, AO
5-13	4	5	40	3 350-3 680	Normal	UA

HMD, hyaline membrane disease
ICH, intracranial hemorrhage
DA, ductus arteriosus
PA, pulmonary artery
AO, aorta
UA, umbilical artery

obtained on vascular tissues of this sample. We obtained the clinical data on two aborted fœtuses of 16 and 18 weeks, in two newborns who died at 26 and 35 weeks of gestation from hyaline membrane disease and one had an additional intracranial hemorrhage. In these four infants we studied tissues of the ductus arteriosus, the pulmonary artery and the aorta and then we studied an additional 8 normal newborns in which we obtained the umbilical artery for the measurements. We could demonstrate biosynthesis of prostaglandins from the C14 arachidonic acid by slices of the above vascular tissues and only would elaborate on (*Table II*). The next studies was similar to the previous one but instead of using C14 arachidonic acid we used C14 prostaglandin NO peroxide PGH^2 and some of the samples were incubated as microsomes not just as slices. The results were similar (*Table III*). A conclusion from this study was that fœtuses as early as 16 weeks gestation possesses signs in enzyme activities for the production of eicosanoids.

Very early in our interest in the EFAs, we postulated that very low birth rate infants will be susceptible to develop rapid onset of EFA deficiency. The reasons are the following: if one look at the composition of infants you can see that 86% is basically water, 1% fat, 8.5% protein and 5% carbohydrates. These infants, if one caculates of a 1 kilogram infant, can see that it contains 110 kcal of non-protein caloric content and because of the low non-protein caloric content, these infants will mobilize fatty acid early in the course for caloric need when the caloric intake is insufficient. The second factor is that the caloric expenditure for very low birth infant is very high. In addition it's very difficult to administer adequate calories to these infants in the form of isotonic glucose and amino-acid solution because excessive fluid is required and hypertonic glucose solution is usually not tolerated well by these infants. Furthermore there are with administration of TPN to these infants the linoleic acid output from adipose tissue is at least partially blocked by increased insulin levels.

In an early study, that we did mid-70s, we measured the plasma fatty acid composition of 5 low birth rate infants with hyaline member disease in the first week of life. They received only a glucose IV solution and we notes in a matter of days a significant drop in the arachidonic acid, an increase in the trienoic acid. The ratio between trienoic/treataenoic exceeded. 4 in a matter of days in the lowest birth rate

Table II. Biosynthesis of prostaglandins from [1 – ^{14}C] arachidonic acid by slices of human vascular tissues*

Tissues	No. Samples	PGF$_{2\alpha}$	PGE$_2$	6-keto PGF$_{1\alpha}$	T x B$_2$	Arachidonic acid
Fetal						
Aorta	2	0.6-0.7	0.4-0.5	0.9-1.2	(–)	97-98
Pulmonary artery	2	0.1-0.2	0.6-0.8	1.2-1.6	(–)	97-98
Ductus arteriosus	2	0.1-0.12	0.4-0.5	1.2-1.4	(–)	97-98
Neonatal						
Aorta	2	0.6-0.7	0.4-0.5	0.9-1.0	(–)	97-98
Pulmonary artery	2	0.1	1.2-1.4	0.8-1.0	(–)	97-98
Ductus arteriosus	2	0.1	1.2-1.6	0.4-0.8	(–)	97-98
Umbilical artery	4	0.6 ± 0.06	0.4 ± 0.02	0.6 ± 0.02	0.5 ± 0.01	97.8 ± 0.2

* Values represent the range or (X ± SEM) of the percent of total radio-activity recovered from the incubation medium.
(–) values not detected.

Table III. Biosynthesis of prostaglandins from [1 – ^{14}C] PGH$_2$ by slices and/or microsomes of human vascular tissues*

Tissues	Slices or microsomes	No. samples	PGF$_{2\alpha}$	PGE$_2$	6-keto PGF$_{1\alpha}$	T × B$_2$	Residue
Fetal							
Aorta	S	1	10.0	12.0	6.0	(–)	72.0
Pulmonary artery	S	1	14.0	9.0	7.0	(–)	70.0
Ductus arteriosus	S	1	6.0	7.0	12.0	(–)	75.0
Neonatal							
Aorta	S	1	6.0	10.0	16.0	(–)	68.0
Pulmonary artery	S	1	14.0	8.0	6.0	(–)	72.0
Ductus arteriosus	S	1	10.0	8.0	12.0	(–)	70.0
Umbilical artery	M	5	11.5 ± 2.5	3.6 ± 3.0	17.0 ± 3.0	3.5 ± 1.0	64.4 ± 2.8

* Single values and (X ± SEM) represent the percent of total radio-activity recovered from the incubation medium.
(–) Values not detected.

infants who was about 700 g; it took between 2 and 3 days to achieve this ratio (*figure 3*). Now these are biochemical changes in the blood and later on studies demonstrated that in these infants it correlated very well with deficient tissue level of EFA.

Until about 10 years ago researchers and clinicians were more interested in the question of prevention and treatment of EFA deficiency rather than thinking nothing about the question of excessive administration of EFA. We were interested in this question and conducted 3 studies, in the first one we compare multiple tissue fatty acid composition of phospholipids in 2 groups of infants. The control infants were

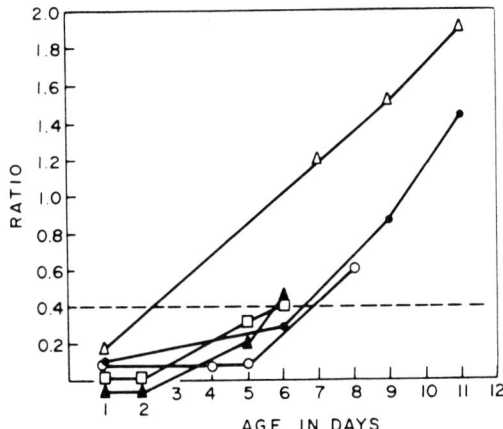

Figure 3. Ratio of Δ-5,8,11-eicosatrienoic acid to arachidonic acid in plasma phospholipids during fat-free diet. Dotted line signifies normal ratio. Open and solid triangles, open and solid circles, and open square each represent a different neonate (from Friedman et al).

infants who died between 4 and 6 months of age from sudden infant death syndrome. These infants were fed either human milk or based-milk formula in which the linoleic acid content was between 5% and 10% of caloric intake. The second group of infants who were on prolonged TPN including parenteral fat emulsion intralipid and then succumbed and we had access to their tissues. We observed that the sum of linoleic acid and arachidonic acid is similar in both these tissues in the control group. In the infants who received TPN and intralipid we noted a significantly increased level of the linoleic acid with a concomitant decrease of the arachidonic acid. We thought that this could result from competition on a esterification and storage of these fatty acids in tissue phospholipid.

The second part of this study was to compare the urinary excretion of the prostaglandin E^1 and E^2 metabolites or PGE-M is 3 groups of infants. There was control infants who were a twelfth of them in which we established, baseline, there was a group of infants who we documented EFA deficiency and group of infants treated using TPN and intralipid intravenously. After the recovery from the deficiency state, the prostaglandin metabolites returned to a control level and then there is a group of infants who we measured the PGE-M before the administration of intralipids and following prolonged adminstration of intralipids and to our astonishment you have level of PGE-M following the prolonged administration of intralipids was similar to that seen in infants with EFA deficiency (*figure 4*). The third studies which I'll just present very briefly because of time was measuring platelet aggregation in infants with EFA deficiency and infants who had received intralipid for prolonged period of time (*figure 5*). In both we found the platelet aggregation was decreased and in further studies we measured the platelet's level of arachidonic acid which was diminished it was decreased a release of C14 arachidonic acid following aggregation and was decreased thromboxine B2 which is a stable metabolite of thrombosine A2 following the aggregation pattern. Thank you for your attention.

Essential fatty acids

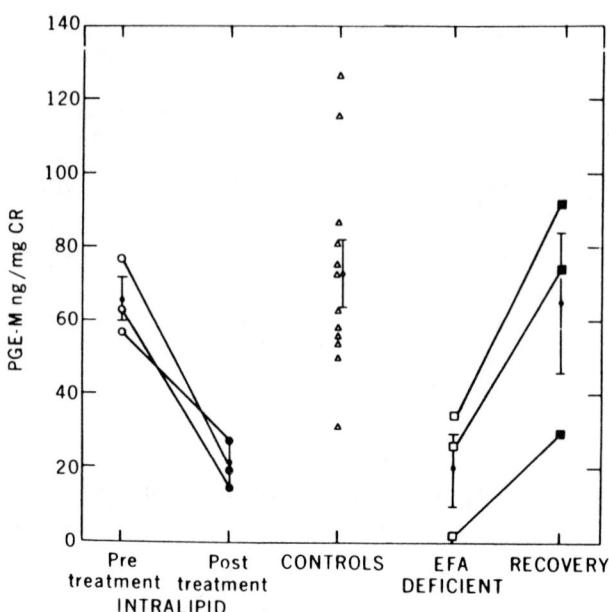

Figure 4. Comparison of the urinary excretion of PGE-M expressed as nanograms per mg urinary creatinine among three groups of infants : (1) infants pre- and post-treatment with Intralipid®; (2) thriving neonates (controls); and (3) infants with EFA deficiency and upon recovery. (From Friedman and Frolich, with permission).

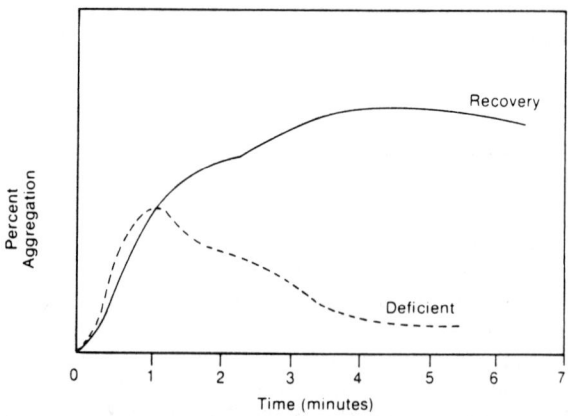

Figure 5. Platelet aggregation patterns at 5.0 µM adenosine 5′-diphosphate during deficient period and ten days after feeding (recovery period).

Summary

The effects of dietary variation in linoleic acid content on tissue phospholipid composition, on the biosynthesis and turnover of prostaglandin E (measured as its major urinary metabolites, PGE-M), and on platelet aggregation were studied in three groups of infants. Group I was comprised of infants with essential fatty acid deficiency; group II infants received linoleic acid (Intralipid R); and group III included the control infants. Infants in group I demonstrated significantly impaired platelet aggregation and disaggregation and a significant decrease in PGE-M excretion when compared to control infants or upon recovery from EFA deficient state. Platelet aggregation and release of thromboxane B2 were similar between groups I and II. Prolonged administration of linoleic acid to sick infants resulted in the incorporation of linoleate into the plasma, platelets, red blood cells, and tissue phospholipids with a concomittant decrease in the arachidonate. PGE-M excretion was similar in infants of groups I and II but significantly lower when compared to control infants. It is concluded that the dietary intake of linoleate has to be carefully monitored, since it may affect platelet function and PGE biosynthesis and turnover. In addition, sick infants may benefit from a balanced dietary intake of linoleate and arachidonate.

Discussion

Dr Bourre: Thank you very much, any question or comment?

Dr Adam: I think it's very interesting, the data on the prostaglandin formation during intralipid administration, you replenish those infants with intralipids in EFA deficiency; you get an increase of PGE-M but if you give it for a prolonged time, you see a decrease of the PGE-M and for me that means 2 things, either the amount of linolenic acid present in intralipid may be transformed to eicosapentanoic acid which is a strong inhibitor of prostaglandin formation and which might be relevant in those infants, because actually as you showed the desaturating process in infants is more active than in adults. That's why I would like to ask you whether you have looked for the formation of eicosapentanoic acid in those infants and whether this increases?

Dr Friedman: We have measured these fatty acids among the others and we have not seen any statistically significant change. We thought that this could be explained by two mechanisms one decreased a substrate; we have seen that arachidonic acid diminishes in tissue phospholipids and second mechanism which has been demonstrated in in vivo studies with linoleic acid is upon the release of fatty acid from phospholipids then with the release of arachidonic acid you have a binding of other fatty acids in this case, it's linoleic acid and it could be a competition between this fatty acids on the cyclo-oxygenase or it could be also a mechanism of inhibition of linoleic acid on the prostaglandin synthesis. There was also other feeding studies on humans and animals to that when there is a replacement of arachidonic acid on tissue phospholipids with other fatty acids then these mechanisms coul operate.

Dr Adam: Don't you think that's a little difference between your two studies in replenishing those infants and there's the same mechanism that you told us working and in the other study where you found the decrease that's not so comparable?

Dr Friedman: I think that the similarities between EFA deficiency and excessive administration of fatty acid is decreased arachidonic acid in tissue phospholipids.

Dr Cunnane: You commented early in your talk about the presence of 23 omega 9 in the serum phospholipids at the various stages 22 to 44 weeks gestation and get the presence of what appeared to be adequate arachidonic acid. And I wonder whether we can establish what the physiological significance of 23 omega 9 in that scenario is, I might put to you that at that stage from my blinkard point of view there's very high levels of copper in the liver in fact it's dropping fairly quickly but towards birth it's very high and it drops then after birth. I think that the copper may be influencing the degree of conversion of oleic to 23 omega 9, one has to debate whether or not the triene/tetraene ratio at that stage in life is a good index of EFA status.

Dr Friedman: That's very interesting. We can certainly find high concentration of 23 omega 9 in cord plasma so every baby who is being born regardless whether he is a premature or full term baby will have this fatty acid in cord plasma. And I postulated I could never I cannot still figure out why this happen and if this is the copper it's a nice solution but we have to do more measurements. The infant, the newborn is certainly not copper deficient because he is receiving enough copper from the mother unless the mother is deficient.

Prof Navarro: It's about your data on prostaglandins and when you compare the effect of intralipids and the effect of the recovery of fatty acid deficiency. And I want to ask you what about the recovery, recovery was done by giving them some linoleic acid or spontaneous?

Dr Friedman: The recovery from EFA deficiency was achieved either by intralipid parenteral fat emulsion or by enteral nutrition.

Prof Navarro: And so the comparison with the intralipid effect, a paradoxical effect, you can explain it only about the amount?

Dr Friedman: The effect of intralipid as opposed to the control group was the excessive amount of linoleic aid which was calculated to be 20% of caloric intake.

Dr Lindohlm: I have a very short question, it's also about the treatment with and without intralipid and the development of EFA deficiency. How long time did it take before you developed EFA deficiency and how long time did it take before they recovered?

Dr Friedman: I'm sorry on which study?

Dr Lindohlm: The last, one of the last, the prostaglandin PGE-M study.

Dr Friedman: The prostaglandin was a long study, we used intralipid at least 6 weeks of intralipid administration and the recovery from excessive administration we did not use the recovery was from the EFA and I cannot recall now whether, how long after the recovery we did I but we certainly demonstrated the recovery at least in serum in plasma that the EFA returned to normal values.

Prof Ghisolfi: Did you have a correlation in your patients between platelet fatty acid contents and platelet aggregation?

Dr Friedman: Yes, but because of limitation of time I didn't bring the slide with me but in infants the initial studies which we did was measure platelet aggregation during EFA deficiency, this we did even before the thromboxane was found and we presented it in the international congress of prostaglandins in Florence. I think it was in 1975. In these studies we did show as I mentioned lastly that there was diminished arachidonic acid in platelet phospholipids, there was diminished release of C14 arachidonic acid with aggregation and decrease thromboxane B^2.

Dr Bourre: And continuing this question, do you have any ideas, do you have some changes in the level of the cholesterol content in the platelets for instance or in any tissue, because if changing the fatty acids then you can control the fluidity by increasing or decreasing the cholesterol content for instance?

Dr Friedman: Yes, we thought about it we did not measure cholesterol. The only measurement we measured is the platelet phospholipid, we are very limited in small infants with the amount of blood that we can draw for these studies and we did not do it.

Dr Ekman: I would like to go back to the study where you showed the decrease in PGE with intralipid. Do you think that observation could be an indices for including let's say gammalinolenic acid into intralipid?

Dr Friedman: We have suggested earlier that perhaps even arachidonic acid as more quantity should be included with intralipid but I don't know any more, I have no solution for this because administration of arachidonic acid to humans has noted to have some side effects and I'm not sure that in sick infants we should include arachidonic acid intravenously.

Dr Bourre: You have to choose the way and on which molecule you inject arachidonic acid, the best way to kill an animal is to inject arachidonic acid including in the brain, you have a huge brain œdema for instance.

Dr Eckman: I would just like to comment this, I think human breast milk has a certain amount of gammalinolenic acid in it.

Dr Friedman: Yes but breast milk has certain amount of gammalinolenic acid and it also has some arachidonic acid.

Dr Eckman: So therefore I think human breast milk has a pattern, it could be a potential idea.

Dr Friedman: I don't know, I think that intravenous administration of EFA in this case it's pharmacologic, it may act differently than enteral nutrition.

Dr Cunnane: In response to the question that you've just raised you still have to make arachidonic acid from GLA and the infant, I think would be able to do that. In adults there's no evidence that you can in fact convert even GLA to arachidonic acid; so I don't think you're any further ahead by putting GLA into the system if you want to get two series prostaglandins out the other end.

Dr Friedman: Yes.

Dr Messing: And just to know a bit more about the toxicity of arachidonic acid, how it acts as you mentioned just in your discussion.

Dr Friedman: Then he pointed that it is acting as being injected in a free form not necessary fat form, so the way it acts I don't know.

Chairman: You have some comment?

Dr Bourre: Well, intravenously one explanation could be thromboxane formation but there are many other possibilities.

Dr Adam: There has been some studies on arachidonic acid given orally in doses of 6 g per day and this study had been cut off within 2 weeks because great formation of thromboxane was noted and the platelet aggregation increased tremendously, so intravenous arachidonic acid is metabolised just the same way and it increases thromboxane with a sequelae of increased pulmonary pressure and platelet aggregation.

Dr Messing: In what form you give arachidonic acid in this experiment you've just mentioned?

Dr Adam: Methyl arachidonic acid.

Dr Bourre: Do you think there is some net transfer through the placenta between the mother and the fœtus for DHA and arachidonic acid or could you speculate if there is some activity in delta 6, delta 5, delta 4 desaturases because there are some differences apparently according to the species, so the only way to know in human could be the stable isotopes for instance, do you think it's possible to decide?

Dr Friedman: Either stable isotopes or isolated placenta perfusion and this has been done years ago in New York. They did it early 60 s or late 50 s. They perfused isolated human placenta and found out that there was a transfer of fatty acids from the mother's side to the fœtus and from the fœtus to the maternal side of the placenta. However using this type of preparation is not ideal because there's a lot of leaking, capillary leaking and the results that you obtain is not accepted totally as correct, stable isotope of course is an excellent tool to answer you question but I don't know if any studies have been done.

Dr Koletzko: There was a paper published last year "Contributions to Gynecology and Obstetrics" by M. Crawford's group who did that with radio actively bought fatty acids and what he showed basically in the perfused human placenta. What he showed basically confirmed the early data that had already proposed that there is a selective maternal fœtal transfer of long chain polyunsaturated metabolites and they also provided data that showed that there is a selective incorporation into the phospholipids. When you look at arachidonic acid for example in maternal plasma and then in placenta phospholipids and in fœtal phospholipids there is a marked increase of the placenta activity where as that is not the case for linoleic acid. So the question that arises from this study is why does nature have an obviously energy requiring process to provide the fœtus in utero with long chain polyunsaturated metabolites across the concentration barrier? My assumption would be that nature would not use an energy requiring process without any sense.

Dr Friedman: Well, in the case of linoleic acid it's not a course it's a course gradient concentration it's not opposite, the linoleic acid in the fœtus is much lower than the mother's so, the long chain are the opposite, but this is the reason we assume that the long chain could be increased because of synthetic activities in the fœtus or combined with preferential transfer.

Chairman: So you have to decide also in terms of gradient where are these molecules because in fact you can have a difference in terms of concentration but only part of these molecules let's say such lipoproteins are actually used, so in fact it is against a gradient but only part of the pool is actually moving and used afterwards.

Dr Koletzko: I'm just a little puzzled now with your last comment, I think that's a very important comment that you proposed because the early studies that you Dr. Friedman have just cited assume that fatty acids were transported across the human placenta by passive diffusion of free fatty acids and they could show that there is a linear correlation between the chain lengths of saturated fatty acids and the placenta transfer and the longer the fatty acid the smaller the transfer, however that holds not true anymore for unsaturated fatty acids, linoleic acid for example is 18. Carbon atoms is transferred at the same rate as palmitic acid for 16 carbon atoms. In other words there must be some other mechanisms and I think what you're saying is very true there is selective binding for example of materna lipid fraction of lipoproteins, phospholipids and they may be transferred across the placenta. The other question of course is where do these healthy P long chain polyunsaturates come from, there was one paper I think from Chambaz and co-workers in Paris that looked for delta 5 desaturase activity in human placenta in mid trimester and they found that there was virtually no activity, very low, suggesting that whereas chain elongation is possible, suggesting that a placenta can synthesise non essential fatty acids but it cannot synthesize arachidonic acid from the precursors and you also know that the newborn infant and the premature infant has a very low capacity, so we basically have to conclude that these fatty acids are coming from the mother.

Dr Friedman: Yes, but in fact the model suggesting that the free form is the only way to get this fatty acid being transported is not so simple. So it's not clear whether we can actually say that they are transported first in the free form according to the chain lengths, according to the number of the saturation which means according to the fluidity differences and the last point is on which molecules, on which proteins these fatty acids are bound because they are potent detergents they can kill the cell very rapidly so are they bound to fatty acide by a binding protein in the free form, or something else ?

Chairman: May I just comment on your remarks? You pointed out to a very important area now of investigation with the correlation between maternal nutrition during pregnancy and the status of the fatty acids in the fœtus. And I don't know, actually there is controversial report in the literature whether in fact there is any correlation between maternal nutrition and the status of EFAs in the fœtus. Have you any report on it, any investigation in this area?

Dr Bourre: Well, I would absolutely agree with you that this is an important question that has to be addressed more in detail.

Chairman: So, maybe I am wrong but I read that the half life of the fatty acid in the adipose tissue is somewhat many months which means that if fatty acids which are used by the fœtus through the mother has been eaten by the mother many months before the pregnancy.

Dr Bourre: So the nutrition of the mother do not include the nutrition just during the pregnancy, it means those fatty acids which has been used which has been fed one year before it can be used by the fœtus, that right?

Dr Friedman: Well, I think the maternal stores of EFAs is only good for several months but the question is very important for us as clinicians is not just during the pregnancy but also during lactation. What would be the effect of maternal nutrition during lactation on milk production and this has been shown a good correlation but during pregnancy I am not familiar.

10

Which essential fatty acids should we supply to the parenterally fed newborn infant ?

B. KOLETZKO

Division of Clinical Nutrition, Department of Paediatrics, The Hospital for Sick Children, Toronto, Ontario, Canada

Introduction

Total parenteral nutrition is a well established and widely applied form of therapy for newborn infants (Am Acad Pediatr'83). Fat emulsions are used with considerable benefit for these patients. They allow infusion of a high energy density in an isotonic solution and, thus, providing total parenteral nutrition via peripheral veins. Currently available preparations are rich in linoleic acid (C 18:2n-6, omega-6 family) and their administration can efficiency prevent the occurence of linoleic acid deficiency. However, in recent years we have become more aware of the powerful physiological functions of other essential fatty acids during early life. Alpha-linolenic acid (C 18:3n-3, omega-3 family) may have an important role in the regulation of linoleic acid metabolism [1, 2]. The long-chain metabolites of both linoleic and alpha-linolenic acids seem to be of major physiological importance during early life.

Essential fatty acids and the newborn infant

The nutritional and metabolic state in the neonatal period differs markedly from any other time of life. When considering the role of essential fatty acids for the newborn infant, some special considerations have to be taken into account (*Table I*). Body stores of essential fatty acids are low at birth. White adipose tissue mass is small, and it may be virtually absent in infants of very low birthweight. Moreover, adipose tissue fat of neonates contains mostly non-essential fatty acids that are synthesized by the fœtus from glucose and ketones [3, 4]. The content of linoleic acid is very small because of its limited placental transfer from the mother ot the fœtus

Table I. Essential fatty acids (EFA) and the newborn infant: special considerations

Low body stores of EFA (e.g. in adipose tissue)
High EFA requirements for deposition in rapidly growing tissues
EFA modulate differentiation and function of developing organs (e.g. linoleic acid stimulates intestinal mucosal growth, prostaglandins mediate the closure of the ductus arteriosus Botalli)
Critical time periods for EFA metabolism (e.g. deposition in CNS lipids during the perinatal phase of rapid brain growth, in contrast to a very slow turnover rate later in life)
Impact of postnatal EFA supply on lipid metabolism and atherogenesis later in life? Triggering of metabolic pathways?
Different metabolic and nutritional states in fullterm, premature and intrauterine growth retarded infants.

[5]. In contrast to low endogenous body stores, there are very high essential fatty acid requirements for deposition in the rapidly growing tissues.

In addition to the various physiological effects of essential fatty acids in the mature organism, in infancy they also modulate organ development by their effects on growth, differentiation and function of the tissues. For example, linoleic acid stimulates intestinal mucosal growth and enhances DNA and protein content as well as sucrase activity in the intestine [6]. Prostaglandins that are derived from essential fatty acids have an important role in the regulation of organ differentiation, such as the closure of the ductus arteriosus Botalli during the first days of life.

A further unique feature of this period of life is the existence of critical time periods. The supply and metabolism of essential fatty acids during the perinatal phase of rapid brain growth determines the composition of structural lipids in the central nervous system, which is related to neutral functions [7, 8, 9]. Since brain lipids have a very low turnover rate after infancy, the quality of perinatal fat supply may influence brain composition for the following decades.

It appears possible that the composition of diet after birth may influence lipid metabolism and the occurrence of obesity and atherosclerosis later in life by triggering metabolic pathways [10, 11]. More research and particularly long-term studies are needed to further elucidate this question.

It is important to remember that newborn infants requiring parenteral feeding comprise a quite heterogeneous patient population. The metabolic and nutritional state of infants born at term differs from that of babies with various degrees of prematurity and it is further altered by intrauterine growth retardation. Moreover, essential fatty acid metabolism may be influenced by clinical variables such as the patient's disease, surgical and other interventions. The essentiel fatty acid state of the parenterally fed infant is also closely related to the intake of total energy, glucose, trace elements and tocopherol.

Linoleic acid deficiency

The supply of linoleic acid is essential to prevent a specific deficiency syndrome. Typically, linoleic acid deficiency is a disorder of infancy. It was characterized by George and Mildred Burr (1929) in rats fed a fat-free diet after weaning, from the 20th day of life onwards. It took as long as between two and a half and three

Table II. Symptoms of essential fatty acid deficiency in rats

Failure to thrive, Weight loss
↓ Utilization of dietary energy & nitrogen
Scaly skin lesions (hind feet, tail), hair loss
↑ Transepidermal water loss
Infections, delayed wound healing
Thrombopenia, ↓ Aggregation, anemia
Fatty liver, infertility

months before scaly skin lesions, a failure to thrive and other symptoms (*Table II*) became apparent. These symptoms do not ocur when the deficient diet is introduced after the animal has reached maturity. Similarly, deficiency symptoms were not observed in a healthy human adult after consumption of a fat-free diet for 6 months [12]. The healthy adult obviously can cover his essential fatty acid requirements for a long period of time by utilizing the considerable reserves that are stored in the body's fat depots.

Human neonates fed with a low fat milk develop clinical signs of deficiency, such as a failure to thrive and skin changes, within two to three months [13]. In contrast to the rather slow development of deficiency symptoms in orally fed infants, a very rapid occurrence of the linoleic acid deficiency syndrome within one to two weeks has been observed in newborn infants receiving fat-free intravenous alimentation (*figure 1*) [14, 15]. Continuous infusion of a high glucose load can lead to

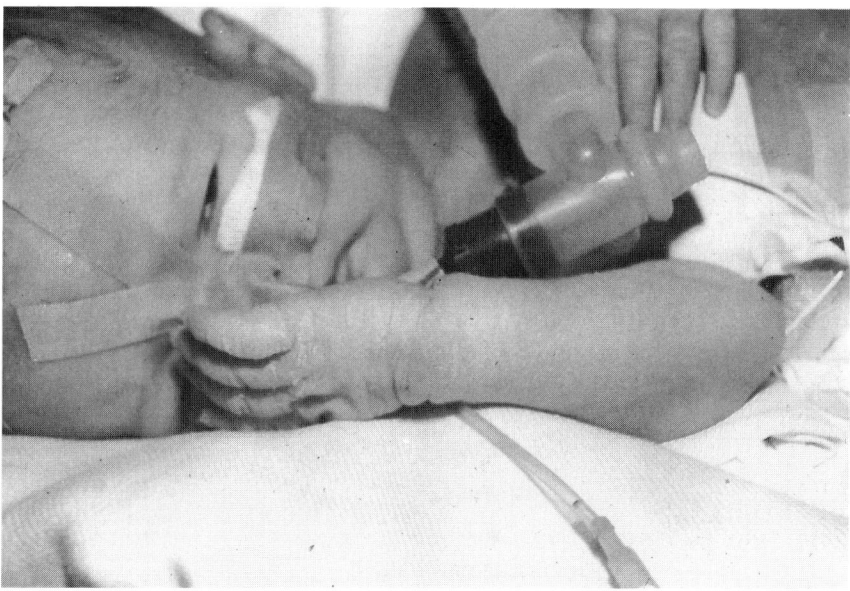

Figure 1. Skin changes in a newborn infant with linoleic acid deficiency after 8 days of fat-free parenteral alimentation. Reproduced with permission from Koletzko, Aktuell Endokrinol Stoffwechsel 1986; 7:18-27.

high insulin levels that prevent adipose tissue lipolysis and, thus, the liberation of linoleic acid from endogenous stores. The deficiency syndrome does not occur when fat emulsions containing linoleic acid are added to the infusion regimen.

Long-chain polyunsaturated fatty acids

The main dietary essential fatty acids, linoleic (C 18:2n-6) and alpha-linolenic (C 18:3n-3) acids, are further desaturated and chain-elongated to long-chain polyunsaturated fatty acids (LCP) by a microsomal enzyme system (figure 2). LCP, such as arachidonic (C 20:4n-6) and eicosapentaenoic (C 20:5n-3) acids, are of physiological importance as precursors for the synthesis of prostaglandins, thromboxanes and leukotrienes (Adam & Wolfram 84). LCP are also essential components of all membrane systems. The LCP content in structural lipids influences membrane fluidity and permeability, the activity of membrane-bound enzymes and the response to electrical excitation (Koletzko 86). During the perinatal phase of rapid brain growth, considerable amounts of LCP are needed for deposition in neural tissues, whereas only traces of linoleic and alpha-linolenic acids are deposited in the membrane lipids of the brain (figure 3) [16-18].

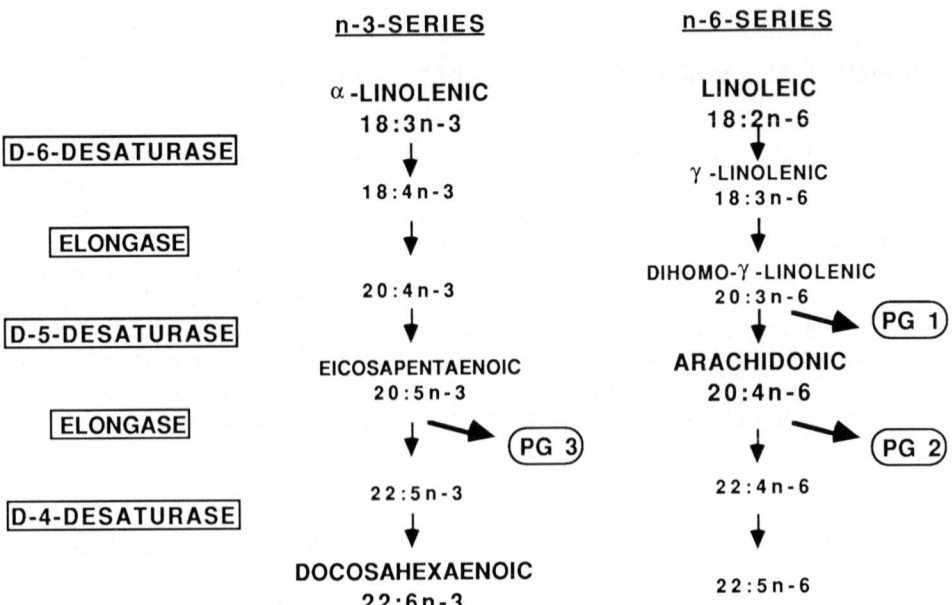

Figure 2. Synthesis of long-chain polyunsaturated fatty acids (LCP) from linoleic and alpha-linolenic acids.

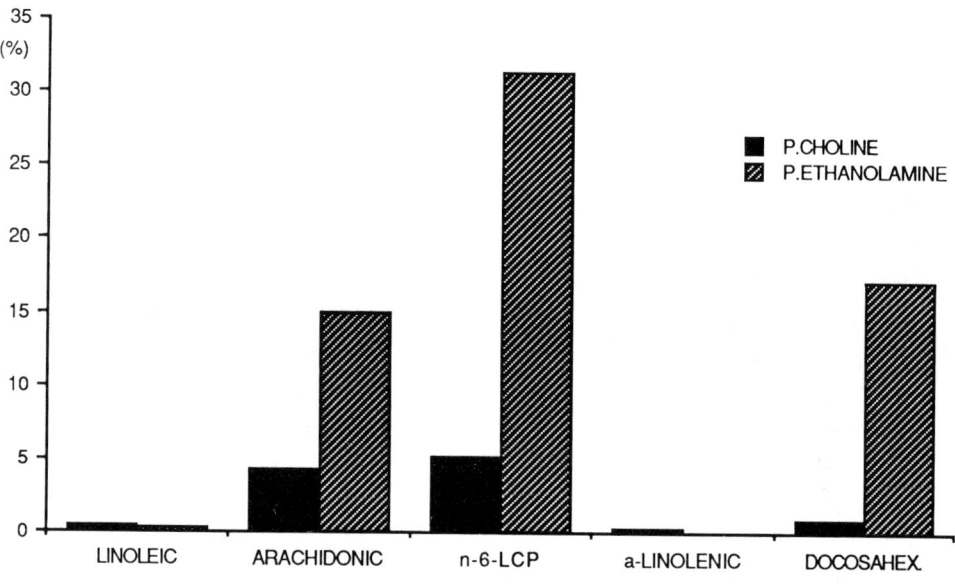

Figure 3. Phospholipid fatty acids of cerebral cortex in the fullterm newborn infant.

Essential fatty acid supply with lipid emulsions

Intralipid is rich in linoleic and alpha-linolenic acids. Only a very minor portion of its essential fatty acid content is contributed by LCP that originate from the phospholipid fraction of the emulsion. LCP of the n-2-series predominate (*figure 4*) (Koletzko et al., unpublished data). Newborn infants have a low capacity to synthesize LCP from linoleic and alpha-linolenic acids, because the activity of the desaturating and chain-elongating enzyme system is low during early life [19]. Human infants who received Intralipid infusions demonstrated high linoleic but low arachidonic acid values in plasma lipid classes [20] plasma lipoprotein lipids [21] and structural lipids of liver and brain [18, 20]. These results question whether the requirements of the neonate can be met by sypplying large amounts of linoleic and alpha-linolenic acids but not of LCP.

Human milk composition as a model for neonatal requirements

Human milk, as the first choice, is recommended as the sole source of food for a healthy infant during the first 4-6 months of life [22]. The composition of human milk is considered a guideline for the desirable nutrient intake in fullterm infants [22]. We studied the lipid composition of mature milk of 15 apparently healthy

Essential fatty acids

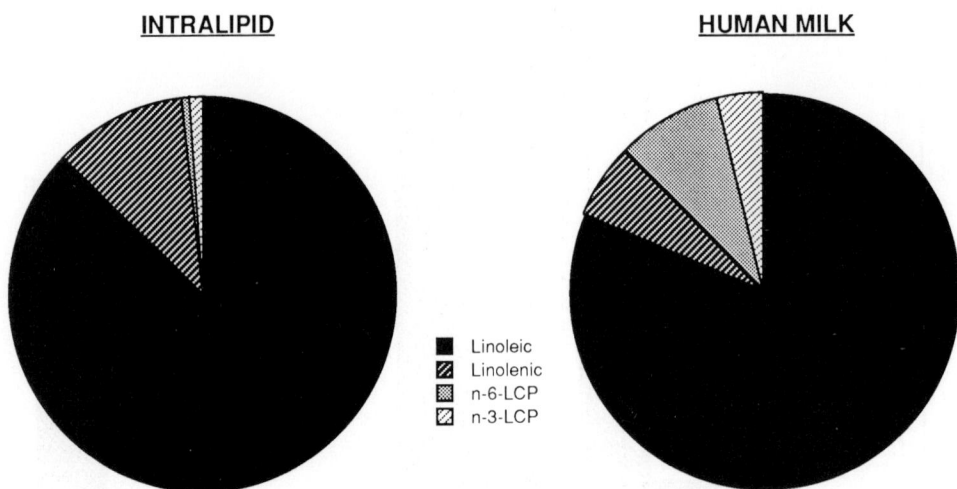

Figure 4. Composition of essential fatty acids in intralipid and human milk.

women, each of whom fully breast fed one infant born at term. Mothers with unusual dietary habits and food fads were excluded by use of a dietary recall protocol. Over a period of 24 hours the mothers manually expressed a sample of milk after each feeding from the breast the infant had nursed on. Hindmilk samples were chosen because they were more convenient to collect for the participating mothers. Also, we have found previously that the fatty acid composition of human milk lipids does not change during nursing [23].

Fatty acid composition of mature human milk

Milk lipids were extracted with methanol/chloroform, fatty acids transesterified with methanolic HCl and their composition analyzed by high-resolution capillary gas-liquid chromatography (*figure 5*) [24]. We separated and quantified, for the first time, 13 different essential fatty acids in human milk lipids (*Table III*). There was a striking degree of inter-individual variation. For example, values for linoleic acid ranged from 5.58 – 21.65% (wt/wt) and those for alpha-linolenic acid from 0.51 – 1.12%. Linoleic acid content of breastmilk has been shown to vary markedly with maternal diet, and thereby with geographic region, cultural traditions and socioeconomic status [24]. It is remarkable that the relative variation of linoleic acid metabolites was smaller than that of linoleic acid. There was no correlation between linoleic or alpha-linolenic acids and their respective LCP-metabolites, indicating that the LCP content of human milk is not regulated by the maternal dietary intake of the two main essential fatty acids. In contrast, a significant correlation was found between n-6, and n-3-LCP in milk (*figure 6*). Milk LCP of both the n-6- and the n-3-series appear to originate primarily from maternal synthesis. The correlation be-

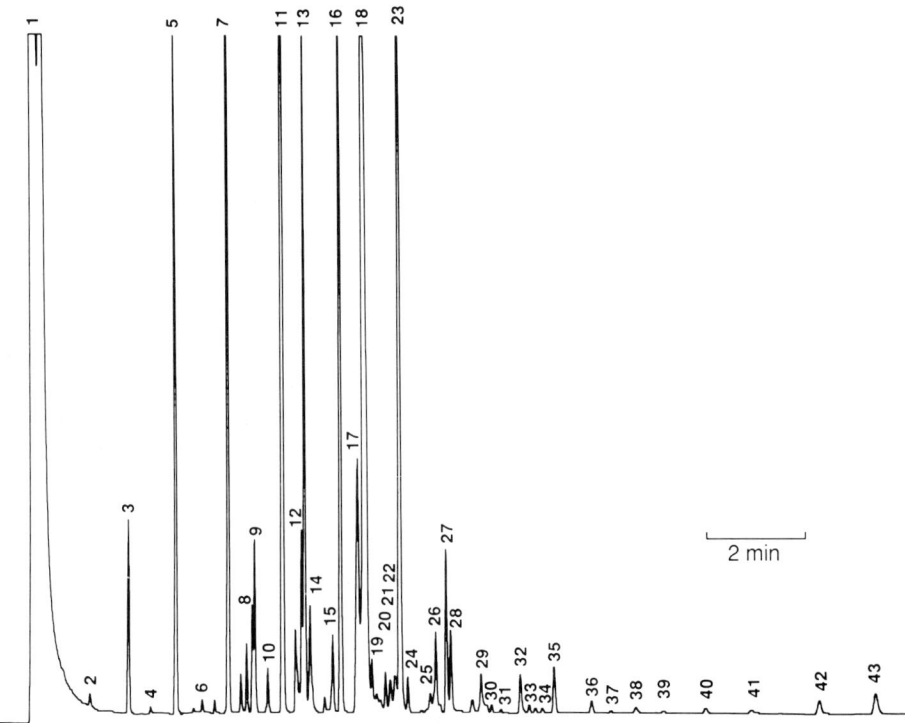

Figure 5. High resolution capillary gas-liquid chromatography of fatty acids in human milk. Reproduced with permission from Koletzko et al., Am J Clin Nutr 1988; 47:954-959.

Table III. Essential fatty acids in mature human milk

Fatty acid	Median	Range
C 18:2n-6	10.76	5.58-21.65
C 18:3n-6	0.16	0.51-1.12
C 20:2n-6	0.34	0.28-0.48
C 20:3n-6	0.26	0.19-0.38
C 20:4n-6	0.36	0.30-0.54
C 22:2n-6	0.08	ND-0.28
C 22:5n-6	ND	ND-0.07
Total n-6	12.26	6.45-22.76
Total n-6-LCP	1.14	0.84-1.73
C 18:3n-3	0.81	0.51-1.12
C 20:3n-3	0.06	ND-0.10
C 20:5n-3	0.04	ND-0.16
C 22:5n-3	0.17	0.11-0.26
C 22:6n-3	0.22	0.15-0.60
Total n-3	1.38	0.84-1.98
Total n-3-LCP	0.51	0.31-1.14

Essential fatty acids

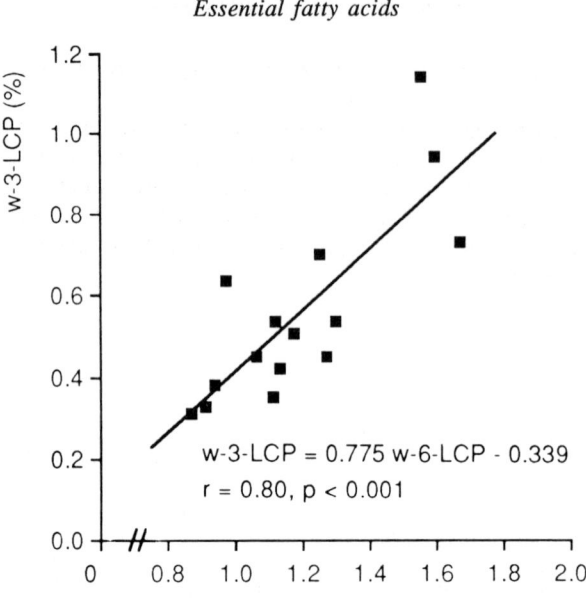

Figure 6. Correlation of omega-6 and omega-3 LCP content in human milk lipids. Reproduced with permission from Koletzko *et al.*, Am J Clin Nutr 1988; 47:954-959.

tween n-6- and n-3-LCP suggests that a common pathway is shared for their synthesis and secretion into milk, whose activity varies between mothers. Therefore, some infants may receive a better supply of both n-6- and n-3-LCP than others. On the other hand, this correlation may also reflect a protective mechanism. The ratio between LCP of the n-6 and n-3 families is kept relatively constant at about 2.3:1, which is similar to that in LCP incorporated into the growing brain. In view of these findings, it appears prudent to avoid unbalanced ratios of n-6/n-3 LCP in parenteral feeding regimens that substitute human milk feeding.

Long-chain polyunsaturated fatty acids : small but beautiful

The LCP content of human milk appears to be small, with arachidonic and docosahexaenoic contributing only 0.4 and 0.2%, respectively, of all milk fatty acids. However, this seemingly small dietary intake has marked effects on the essential fatty acid status of the newborn infant. Preliminary results of a feeding study in premature infants ([21], Koletzko *et al.*, unpublished data) indicate that in infants fed human milk, the content of arachidonic and docosahexaenoic in plasma lipids remains constant during the first three weeks of life. In contrast, feeding of an adapted milk formula that supplies linoleic and alpha-linolenic acid content in amounts similar to human milk, but is devoid of LCP, leads to a marked LCP-depletion of plasma lipids ([21], Koletzko *et al.*, unpublished data). These results indicate that the capacity to synthesize LCP is limited during early life, and that postnatally a dietary LCP supply may be essential to avoid distortion of plasma and membrane lipid composition.

For parenterally fed infants, the development of lipid emulsions with an essential fatty acid composition closer to that of human milk than the products presently available (*figure 4*) could be beneficial. The use of such modified fat emulsions might result in improvements of the infants' essential fatty acid status that may be especially valuable in infants of low and very low birthweight and in infants requiring long-term parenteral feeding.

Références

1. Budowski P., Crawford M.A. (1985) Alpha-linolenic acid as a regulator of the metabolism of arachidonic acid: dietary implications of the ratio, n-6: n-3 fatty acids. *Proc. Nutr. Soc.* 44:221-229.
2. Koletzko B., Mrotzek M., Bremer H.J. (1988) Fatty acid composition of mature human milk in Germany. *Am. J. Clin. Nutr.* 47:954-9.
3. Widdowson E.M., Dauncey M.J., Gairdner D.M.T., Jonxis J.H.P., Pelikan-Filipkova M. (1975) Body fat of British and Dutch infants. *Brit. Med. J.* 1:653-5.
4. Andersen G.E., Christensen N.C., Petersen M.B.V., Johansen K.B. (1987) Fatty acid composition of subcutaneous adipose tissue in mother-infant pairs. *Acta Paediatr. Scand.* 76:87-90.
5. Dancis J., Janssen V., Kayden H.J., Schneider H., Levitz M. (1973) Transfer across perfused human placenta. II. Free fatty acids. *Pediatr. Res.* 7:192-7.
6. Hart M.H., Grandjean C.J., Park J.H.Y., Erdman S.H., Vanderhoof J.A. (1988) Essential fatty acid deficiency and postresection mucosal adaptation in the rat. *Gastroenterology* 94:682-7.
7. Lamptey M.S., Walker B.L. (1976) A possible essential role for dietary linolenic acid in the development of the young rat. *J. Nutr.* 102:86-93.
8. Bourre J.M., Pascal G., Durand G., Masson M., Dumont O., Piciotti M. (1984) Alterations in the fatty acid composition of rat brain cells (neurons, astrocytes, and oligodendrocytes) and of subcellular fractions (myelin and synaptosomes) induced by a diet devoid of n-3 fatty acids. *J. Neurochem.* 43:342-8.
9. Yamamoto N., Saitoh M., Moriuchi A., Nomura M., Okuyama H. (1987) Effect of dietary a-linolenate/linoleate balance on brain lipid composition and learning ability of rats. *J. Lipid. Res.* 28:144-51.
10. Hahn P. (1987) Obesity and atherosclerosis as consequences of early weaning. In: Ballabriga A., Rey J. (eds) Weaning: why, what and when? Raven Press, New York, pp. 93-113.
11. Hamosh M. (1988) Does infant nutrition affect adiposity and cholesterol levels in the adult? *J. Pediatr. Gastroenterol. Nutr.* 7:10-16.
12. Brown W.R., Hansen A.E., Burr G.O., McQuarrie I. (1938) Effects of prolonged use of extremely low-fat diet on an adult human subject. *J. Nutr.* 16:511-24.
13. Von Gröer F. (1919) Zur Frage der praktischen Bedeutung des Nährwertbegriffes nebst einigen Bemerkungen über das Fettminimum des menschlichen Säuglings. *Biochem. Z.* 97:311-29.
14. Friedman Z., Danon A., Stahlman M.T., Oates J.A. (1976) Rapid onset of essential fatty acid deficiency in the newborn. *Pediatrics* 58:650-9.
154. Koletzko B. (1986) Essentielle Fettsäuren. Bedeutung für Medizin und Ernährung. *Aktuell Endokrinol. Stoffwechsel.* 7:18-27.
16. Svennerholm L. (1968) Distribution and fatty acid composition of phosphoglycerides in normal human brain. *J. Lipid. Res.* 9:570-9.

17. Clandinin M.T., Chapell J.E., Leong S., Heim T., Swyer P.R., Chance G.W. (1980) Intrauterine fatty acid accretion rates in human brain: implications for fatty acid requirements. *Early Human Dev.* 4:121-9.
18. Martinez M., Ballabriga A. (1987) Effects of parenteral nutrition with high doses of linoleate on the developing human liver and brain. *Lipids* 22:133-8.
19. Koletzko B., Bremer H.J. (1987) Long chain polyunsaturated fatty acids in infant formulae. *Eur. J. Pediatr.* 146:92.
20. Friedman Z., Frolich J.C. (1979) Essential fatty acids and the major urinary metabolites of the E prostaglandins in thriving neonates and in infants receiving parenteral fat emulsions. *Pediatr. Res.* 13:932-6.
21. Koletzko B., Schmidt E., Bremer H.J., Haug M., Harzer G. (1987) Dietary long chain polyunsaturates for premature infants. *J. Pediatr. Gastroenterol. Nutr.* 6:997-999.
22. ESPGAN Committee on Nutrition (1982) Guidelines on infant nutrition. III. Recommendations for infant feeding. *Acta Paediatr. Scand.* Suppl. 302:1-27.
23. Koletzko B., Mrotzek M., Bremer H.J. (1985) Fat content and cis- and trans- isomeric fatty acids in human fore- and hindmilk. In: Hamosh M., Goldman A.S., eds., Human lactation 2: Maternal and environmental factors. New York, London: Plenum Press, 589-594.
24. Koletzko B., Cunnane S. (1988) Human alpha-linolenic acid deficiency ? *Am. J. Clin. Nutr.* 47:1084-1086.
25. Burr G.O., Burr M.M. (1929) A new deficiency disease produced by the rigid exclusion of fat from diet. *J. Biol. Chem.*, 82:345-67.
26. Adam O., Wolfram G. (1984) Effect of different linoleic acid intakes on prostaglandin biosynthesis and kidney function in man., *Am. J. Clin. Nutr.,* 40:763-70.
27. American Academy of Pediatrics, Committee on Nutrition (1983) Commentary on parenteral nutrition. *Pediatrics,* 71:547-552.
28. Koletzko B., Whitelaw A., Takeda J., Filler R.M., Heim T. (1987) Linoleic acid metabolism in parenterally fed infants. *Pediatr. Res.* 22:232.

Summary

In supply of essential fatty acids is of marked physiological importance in the neonatal period, when body stores are low and requirements are high. Commonly available lipid emulsions can efficiently prevent the occurrence of linoleic acid deficiency. However, these preparations contain only small proportions of long-chain polyunsaturated metabolites (LCP) both of linoleic and alpha-linolenic acids. The infant requires LCP as substrates for prostaglandin synthesis and for tissue and brain growth. Endogenous synthesis of LCP from the main dietary essential fatty acids appears to be low during early life. Parenterally fed infants show reduced LCP values in plasma and tissue lipids in spite of a large precursor supply. The composition of human milk lipids may to some extrent serve as a guideline for neonatal requirements. Human milk contains significant amounts of LCP with a relatively constant ratio of n-6 and n-3 LCP. The development of lipid emulsions with an essential fatty acid composition closer to that of human milk coul be beneficial for parenterally fed infants.

Discussion

Dr Bourre: Thank you very much for this nice presentation. Any questions or comments?

Dr Friedman: I would like to make a comment on the EFA composition of human milk. There have been some studies in third world countries and we have studied this question in detail. When we did the studies on prostaglandins in human milk and you can change the composition of EFAs in human milk with maternal diet and this is not new. You can measure human milk composition in vegetarian mothers where the composition or the per cent of EFAs was markedly increased in human milk in these mothers. But it' very true and it's astonishing to see that usually the linoleic acid was the one to go up but the arachidonic acid is pretty much constant per cent of the fatty acid composition. I do not know what the solution is for this, what's the explanation. Also the breast milk is rich in prostaglandins and maternal diet does not change the composition of prostaglandins in human milk which is another astonishing dilemma, I dont't know how to explain this to you.

Dr Koletzko: Yes I would absolutely agree with that. Diet does change the linoleic acid content of human milk very markedly and you find a lot of variation in studies from different parts of the world and also in studies of different dietary habits for example. In the comparison of vegetarians and non-vegetarians, linoleic acid was increased markedly in the vegetarians whereas arachidonic acid, mean arachidonic acid values in both groups were 4%, there was no influence of vegetarian diet on that and I think that is very striking. Why is that so and could there be some physiological regulation that makes sure that the infant gets and appropriate amount of LCP?

Dr Bourre: One explanation could be that these lipids, these fatty acids are not in the same pool, you have the triglycerides and you have the phospholipids, so you have phospholipids which are actually found in membrane in the milk and these phospholipids probably have polyunsaturated fatty acid whose composition is heavily controlled as in any membrane, in contrast with the triglycerides; so could you tell what is the proportion between those two under normal condition the phospholipids versus the triglycerides for instance?

Dr Koletzko: That's a very good comment. Yes phospholipids of course have also in human milk a such higher content of arachidonic acid and other LCP in percentage composition but the bulk of human milk lipids, 98-99%, is comprised by triglycerides and also if you calculate the absolute amount of LCP, phospholipids actually contribute only a very small portion to the LCP in human milk and most of the LCP actually is found in the triglyceride. If you look at the composition of human milk during nursing compare fore and hind milk, there is a marked change in the phospholipid content, the relative content of phospholipids, but the LCP content is not changed at all so I think phospholipid LCP are not a major factor. They may have a physiological role, we do not know whether they are absorbed or metabolised differently or whether they have other effects.

Dr Cunnane: I accept the point that your making about the uniformity of the arachidonic acid levels regardless of linoleic acid. If you think about it is really has to be that way if you're going to guarantee the fœtal brain, amongst the other organs, but particularly the brain, the right amount of arachidonic acid for its development, because across species we see the same amount of arachidonic acid in the brain regardless whether it's a dow or a rat or a human, arachidonic acid content of the brain is still the same, so evolution has determined over millenia that there is a certain amount that is required and it's not going to be by coincidence that the arachidonic acid and the docosahexanoic acid in the milk are there at a minimal and essentially inflexible amount. The mother has a system to virtually guarantee at her own risk that those be there for the infant whereas linoleic acid is not required by the brain and therefore can afford to be more variable.

Dr Bjerve: Do you have any data on the fatty acid composition of blood lipids of the mothers. Do they reflect what kind of milk they will produce. Can you deduce from the fatty acid composition of let's say plasma phospholipids what kind of milk they will produce. And another question linked to it will you always expect mothers from modern western societies to produce milk high enough in content in all these EFAs, both omega 3s and omega 6s. Because you are analysing human milk and using that as a guideline and there are quite a lot of variations also on the long chain, varies by more than 100%. If your going for the low values will you still be supplying reasonably enough of the long chains.

Dr Koletzko: To answer your first question, we have not looked at the correlation between plasma lipids and milk lipids in this study but this is known that there is a correlation, other studies have shown that previously that of course dietary intake influences plasma lipids and is also correlated to human milk lipids and there is a correlation between the fatty acid or let's say linoleic acid content in plasma lipids. The second question I think I cannot answer presently, as you saw there is an individual variation in the LCP supply to the infant and what is the mechanism of regulation and what is the physiological impact and what is the range of that we do not know. We do know that certain maternal illnesses alter the composition of milk lipids and it may well be possible that in some mothers, the EFA supply with human milk is suboptimal.

Dr Messing: You mentioned that linoleic acid stimulate mycosal growth of intestine and so my question is it different from other saturated or unsaturated fatty acid and how it can act on the mycosal growth of intestinal cells. What is the mechanism of this effect?

Dr Koletzko: There was a very recent paper. They showed that in short gut syndrome if you supply linoleic acid after short gut syndrome you have an increase in DNA and protein content of intestinal causal cell, this is a specific effect of linoleic acid. I think there is no clue as yet on mechanism.

Dr Adam: I'm a little bit puzzled about the relation of omega 6 to omega 3 fatty acids which you have shown as constant with all variations and plasma lipids show a different pattern. So actually the fatty acids you find in the milk are not related to the fatty acid composition of plasma or anything like that. Would you tell me whether this correlation of omega 6 to omega 3 indicates the amount of fat present in the milk or is it correlated to phospholipid content of the milk or anything like that.

Dr Koletzko: I sympathise very much with you when you say you are puzzled, that was exactly my reaction to when I was thinking for a long while what is happening here and I must admit that I'm not quite sure about the answers yet. With regard to the correlation to plasma lipids I said this is true for linoleic acid, for n-6 n-3 LCP it has not been investigated that closely and I should agree with you that is an interesting question what is the mechanism phospholipids in maternal plasma for example related or not. As I said previously it's not the phospholipids in milk it is not correlated to total fat content.

Dr Martinez: If you analyse mature milk all the time, I mean have you analysed colostrum or transitional milk, human milk?

Dr Koletzko: In this study we have focussed on milk samples from the third and fourth month of lactation, that is mature milk. Most investigators define mature milk as milk after six weeks of lactation.

Dr Martinez: Yes because if I understood well you say that the ratio omega 6 to omega 3 of long chain fatty acids keeps constant. Perhaps it could be a little higher first, because at least in the human brain this ratio is going down early in development, could be something interesting.

Dr Koletzko: That's an interestering question yes.

Dr Friedman : To answer the last question we have analysed the human milk composition for fatty acid on the same models, in the first three days of life which represented colostrum and then from up to seven days which was a transitional milk and then mature milk at two weeks of age and there was no changes in the EFAs in these three samples.

Dr Koletzko: Well there's different results. There was another study published in 1983 in the American Journal of Clinical Nutrition who looked closely at the development of the fatty acid pattern during lactation by Harzer and coworker. They in fact found that there is a change with the duration of lactation, but again they did not look at this correlation.

Dr Friedman: There was a change in total fat.

Dr Koletzko: There was a change in the fatty acid composition with the duration of lactation.

Dr Friedman: May be they went over two weeks, we measured the fore milk and the hind milk on the same sample.

Dr Koletzko: Oh I'm sorry.

Dr Friedman: I have another question to you, I am a great promoter of human milk feedings for prematures as well as full term but listening to you can you tell me, how do babies develop normal CNS on cow's milk based formulas only with no supplementation of arachidonic acid?

Pr Koletzko: I do not know whether they develop the normal brain or not. Who has analysed that? I dont't think we have any data on it.

Dr Friedman: We must assume since in western countries in the last 20 or 30 years maybe 60% and over of the population are going on cow's milk based formulas unfortunately but, this is what happens.

Dr Koletzko: Yes but we must also see that there have been a lot of Immunological studies that showed that formula fed infants are in fact at a disadvantage. Formula fed infants over the last two or three decades have a lot of disadvantages over breast fed infants. There's also studies on psychological performance. Of course it's difficult to say what is the factors involved, is it really biochemical factors or some people have suggested it is the different behaviour of the infants because they have to be sort of more patient until they get their milk and therefore this triggers a different behaviour later on in approaching problems that you are so forth patient. I do not know but it is certainly not the case that formula fed infants have the same performance as breast fed infants.

Dr Friedman: Don't understand me wrongly, I'm a great promoter of human milk but still biochemically what happened to these infants who are going just on infant formula without arachidonic acid supplementation?

Dr Koletzko: I can only say that I was very impressed by the correlation that Dr Martinez published. The close correlation between fatty acids in brain and fatty acids in liver and I think that we have to assume that plasma fatty acids are largely the fatty acids synthesized in the liver and that therefore, what we see in plasma and what we see in red blood cells, may really be related to the brain.

Chairman: OK, so in fact, it means that we are not in the best shape as we would have been if having been breast fed but we are not dying. So the very last question.

Dr Cunnane: The brain also has the ability to synthesize arachidonic acid and docosahexanoic acid as is the fœtal liver, the heart and the kidney so that there is not a total absence of a synthetic capacity and whether or not it prefers to get if preformed from the milk is another issue as long as it is available and obviously that's going to take place.

Dr Koletzko: But that's not data from the human.

Dr Cunnane: We don't know that human liver, human brain synthesizes arachidonic acid no.

Dr Koletzko: We know that the rat has a much higher capacity of synthesizing long chain polyunsaturates than the human and we do not know whether the human brain, the noenate brain is capable of synthesizing.

Dr Cunnane: Well these are different by degree but are not likely to be different like a total absence versus the presence in another species so we don't know the degree to which the brain can synthesize it, but it's evident in the absence of its being in the milk that maybe we don't have optimal levels of it in the brain but certainly there's going to be some there so synthetic capacity has to exist.

Chairman: So I suggest you continue this nice discussion tonight when enjoying the omega 3 fatty acid you will get in your dinner.

11

Essential fatty acids, parenteral nutrition and the developing human

M. MARTINEZ

Hospital Infantil Vall d'Hebron, Passeig de la Vall d'Hebron, 08035, Barcelona, Spain

The extraordinarily high proportion of very long polyunsaturated fatty acids in membrane phospholipids, especially in those of the central nervous systems is remarkable. Among the polyunsaturated fatty acids, docosahexanoic acid as you know and arachidonic acid are the mere fatty acids, especially in phosphatidylethanolamine and phosphatidylcholine. Therefore the supply of these fatty acids to the developing human must be very important seeing. It has been demonstrated that delta 6 desaturase is not very active in the human infant. However for many years now, formulas manufactured for oral adminsitration and also for parenteral nutrition, are very rich in linoleic acid and most of them very poor in alphalinolenic acid. Besides there is very little content of long polyunsaturated fatty acids in most of these formulas. Alphalinolenic acid has even been considered as essential for many years, since Tinoco and co-workers work and some others. However it seems extraordinary that the high proportion of docosahexanoic acid in the retina and in the nervous system in general does not mean something. So we have been very worried for a long time on this problem.

We studied a group of 18 neonates with different gestational ages for the ethanolamine and choline phosphoglycerides, the fatty acid patterns of these two phospholipids during development, during normal development. These children died immediately or during the 24 or 48 hours of life and had not been fed yet. These newborns were appropriate, the weight of these newborns was appropriate for gestational age. The nutritional status was very good and they died during the first hours either because of prematurity or acute respiratory disease.

Since I think it's in order to make things more simple, I would like to centre my discussion upon the two main polyunsaturated fatty acids, docosahexanoic acid and arachidonic acids. But the main changes in the two tissues were aware and increasing docosahexanoic acid of a parabolic type, a decrease of arachidonic acid with gestational age in both phospholipids and a quite linear decrease of oleic acid. But as I say I prefer to discuss only what makes reference to these two polyunsaturated fatty acids because after all we are discussing about the possibility of nutrition paradox in these polyunsaturated fatty acids.

You can see that in the liver (*figure 1*) ethanolamine phosphoglycerides, you have parabolic increase; so that up to 30 weeks there is almost no increase and then there is a really abrupt increase after this age. This is in the liver and you can see that at the beginning, it's about 10% and then at the end of gestation, it's something over 20 which means very similar to the brain levels. So there is just before then a very rapid increase. In the brain (*figure 2*) the increase is also par-

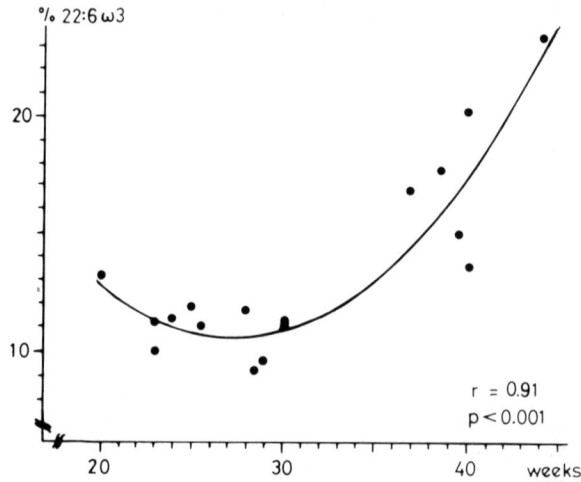

Figure 1. Docosehexaenoic acid percentage in liver ethanolamine phosphoglycerides (EPG) and gestational age (weeks).

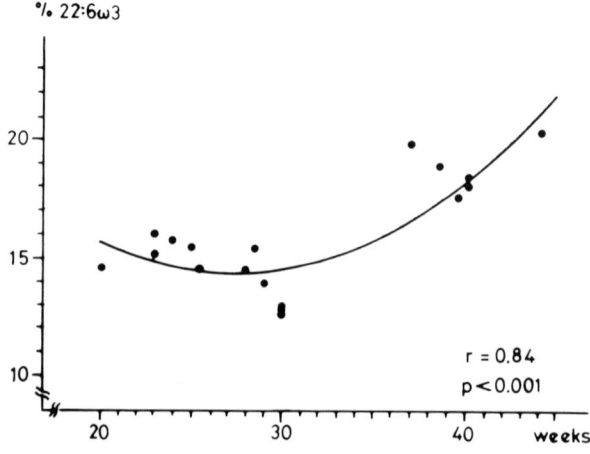

Figure 2. Docosahexaenoic acid percentage in brain ethanolamine phosphoglycerides (EPG) and gestational age (weeks).

abolic and you see that the increase is not so fast, because the initial levels are higher, 15% but the final levels are about the same. I prefer to present you with these real data instead of the groups data which have been published so that you can see case by case. Then if we look at the arachidonic acid percentage in ethanolamine phosphoglycerides you have a decrease also of a parabolic type and levels were of about 30% before 30 weeks and then there is a precipitious decrease after this time in the arachidonic acid profile in the liver (*figure 3*). In the brain there is also a decrease of these fatty acids (*figure 4*). This decrease is almost linear and you see also arachidonic acid goes down with gestational age.

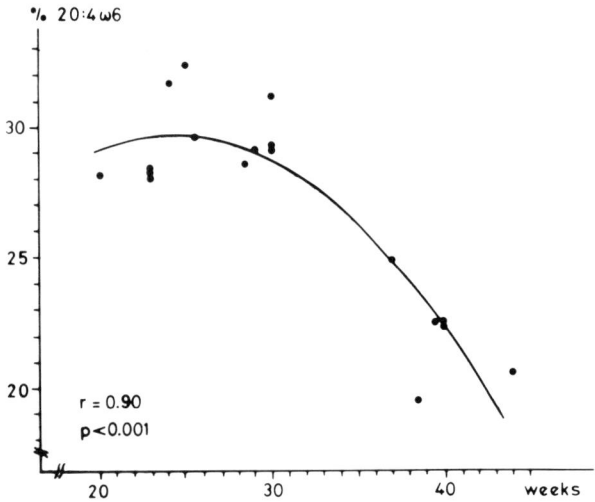

Figure 3. Arachidonic acid percentage in liver phosphoethanolamine (EPG) and gestational age.

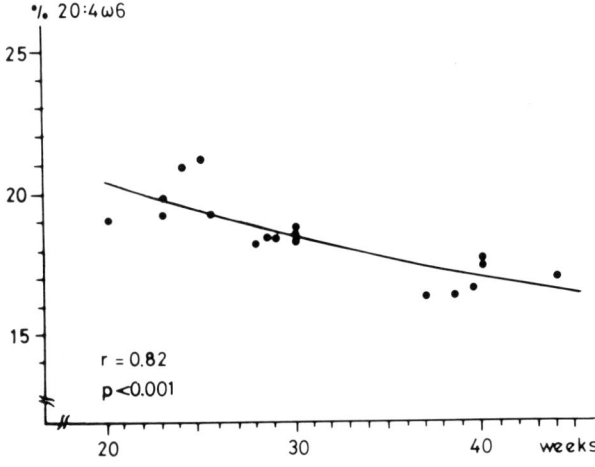

Figure 4. Arachidonic acid percentage in brain phosphoethanolamine (EPG) and gestational age.

Essential fatty acids

So, these two fatty acids the, docosahexanoic acid and arachidonic acid, are quite opposite in the profile, one goes up and the other goes down during this time.

We tried to correlate case by case the changes of these two fatty acids in ethanolamine phosphoglycerides of the liver and brain, and we found that really there was a positive correlation because the increase was in this case very similar although the curve rose faster in the liver as I have shown before. So you get that when we correlate case by case the levels of docosahexanoic in liver and brain, you get a positive correlation in this fatty acid which is increasing. And in the other which is decreasing because it is decreasing more or less about the same rate in the two organs you get also a positive correlation when you plot the brain values against the liver values of these fatty acids.

In order to emphasise the different profile of these two fatty acids in both tissues, we tried also case by case to plot the docosahexanoic levels against the arachidonic levels and as you can see there is really in the liver a negative correlation because there is an inverse relationship within certains limits. And you can see that between 20 and 30 weeks the decrease is very fast and this tends to level off (*figure 5*). In the case of the brain when we tried to correlate these two fatty acids (*figure 6*) you get also a parabolic profile but the decrease is only from 16% of arachidonate to 20% of arachidonate you get negative correlation and then there is a tendency to go up. We don't know that this means because we need more basis of ages, older ages. This is all prenatal, that means that this is development intra-uterus.

Then we were very interested in looking at what happens in children having received TPN, with intralipid. Intralipid is the most widely used infusion, we have been using it for many years in our hospital. As you know very well it has over 50% of linoleic acid and compared to other perfusions, you have a high level also

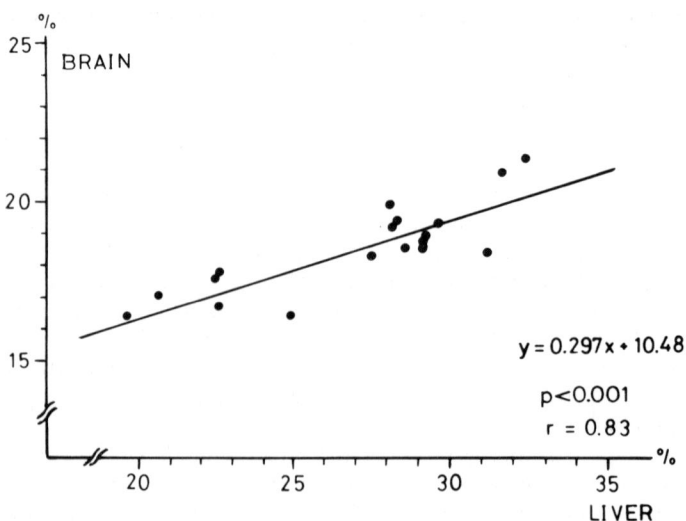

Figure 5. Brain against liver percent values of arachidonic acid in ethanolamine phosphoglycerides in newborns in function of gestational age.

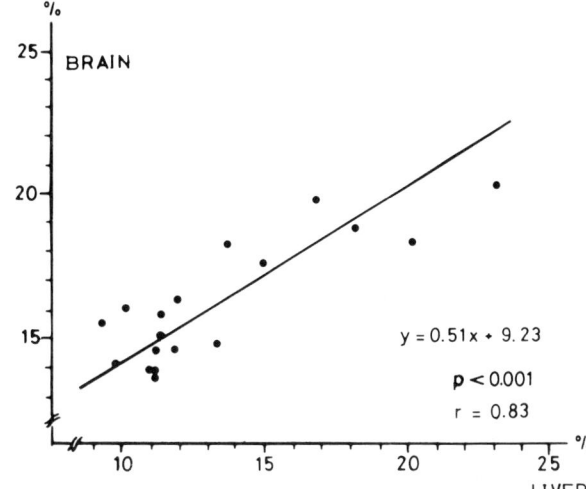

Figure 6. Brain against liver percent values of docosahexaenoic acid in ethanolamine phosphoglycerides in newborns in function of gestational age.

of linolenate, relatively high with according to the repeated batches, I have been studying the ratio of linoleate to alphalinolenate is between 7 and 8. So theoretically, this should cause no trouble at all. We studied these children, these children were a group of children with surgical problems. They died shortly after birth because of complications. The maximum they lived was 15 days and they have received TPN for between 4 and 14 days, 12 days as a maximum. So they received TPN for a very short time. The total fat intake was around for the 7 g fat, ranging from the 29 to 90 as a maximum. We wanted to look at the same parameters and I am going to show you again only the two main polyunsaturates in ethanolamine phosphoglycerides which are the main unsaturated phospholipids. To simplify. You have here the per cent value of linoleate, arachidonate and docosahexanoic acid in choline phosphoglycerides (*figure 7*), which are not much unsaturated but in this case I want to show you these phospholipids because there are indeed very significant changes also in these phospholipids. So you have linoleic which has increased more than double, the value in the controls in liver, you have the docosahexanoic which is about half the normal value of the controls in the children having received TPN and arachidonate in this case is significantly increased. I must emphasise that this is a standard deviation, not a standard error, so this is very significant. When we look to the most unsaturated phospholipid you have here that linoleic acid has increased three times the control values in the children having received TPN, whereas docosahexanoic acid despite the very short period they have received intralipid is decreased to half the control values and this is very significant because there is no overlapping of standard deviation. In this case, I mean in ethalonamine phosphoglycerides (*figure 8*), there is no significant variation whatsoever in the per cent values of the liver arachidonate.

Well as this indicated that the excess of linoleic supplied didn't serve to elongate this fatty acid and to produce more arachidonic acid because either it was unchanged or it was decreased in choline phosphoglycerides, we tried to study an index which was expressed the desaturation elongation of linoleic acid. You have all the main products of linoleic in the numerator and linoleic acid in the denominator (*figure 9*).

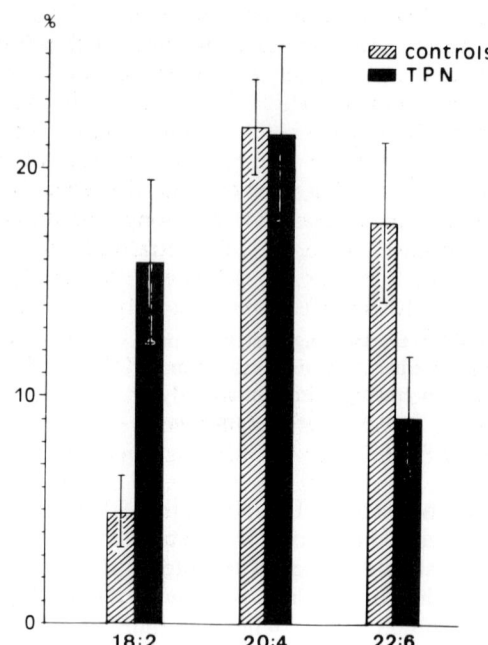

Figure 7. Per cent values of linoleate, arachidonate and docosahexaenoic acid in liver choline phosphoglycerides.

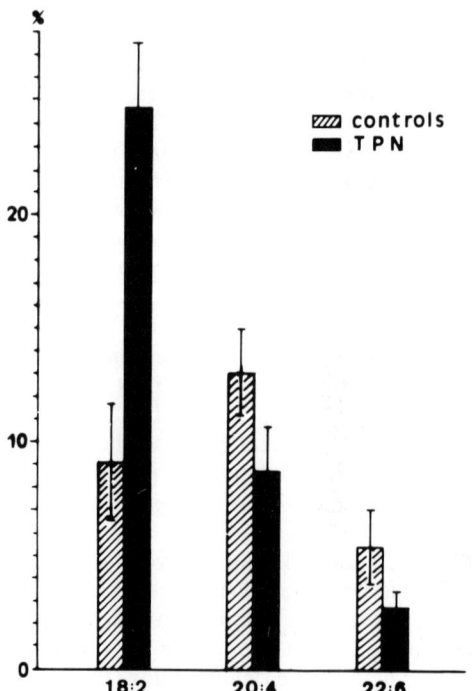

Figure 8. Per cent values of linoleate, arachidonate and docosahexaenoic acid in liver ethanolamine phosphoglycerides.

So this is an index which is good to study the desaturation elongation of this fatty acid. And we can see that it should be expected in liver EPG you have a very important decrease of elongation of this fatty acid. This decrease in the elongation of linoleate is also very important in liver CPG in choline phosphoglycerides but in the brain in which I must say we could not find any change for the moment probably because these children had been taking intralipid for a short time, the only change we could find was an increase of linoleic acid not accompanied by an increase of the longer members. So when we used this index, we could find a very significant decrease of the elongation/desaturation in the brain. I cannot say what could have happened if the intralipid would have last longer, I cannot say of course. I think, these results indicate quite clearly that a large assess of linoleic acid has some adverse effects on long polyunsaturated fatty acid formation, since in the first place it is so to sat useless to its own family because it does not produce more longer omega 6 polyunsaturated fatty acids, rather it seems to inhibit their formation as some workers have found, and I have found in choline phosphoglycerids. Then in the second place, it has been damaging to the omega 3 family because of enzymatif competition for the desaturase systems. This mechanism is very understandable for preparations that have a large access of linoleic acid but have almost no linolenic acid. But why is it that intralipid which has a correct linoleic to alphalinolenic ratio

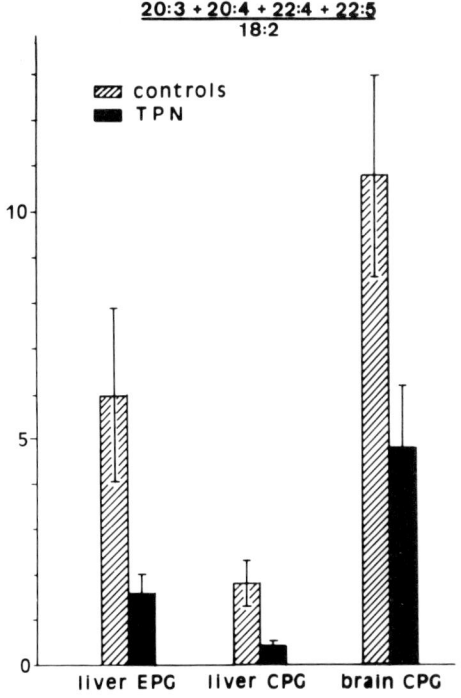

Figure 9. n-6 higher homologues fatty acids/linoleic acid ratio in liver ethanolamine phosphoglycerides, liver choline phosphoglycerides, and brain choline phosphoglycerides, in control and TPN infants.

reduce the docosahexanoic content of tissue so much? I would like you to think about this. Personally I cannot find any other explanation than an access of precursors is inhibiting in a way the formation of the longer polyunsaturated fatty acids. It should be very nice to try to prepare some new products which has less precursors and more long polyunsaturated fatty acids. Yesterday was discussed that too much polyunsaturated could be damaging, it is true but I am just proposing to use the right portion. As Dr Koletzko pointed out yesterday I think we should imitate human milk as much as possible. I've never understood why 50% of linoleic acid should be used because there is no tissue in the body with 50% of linoleic acid. In the blood normally for a person who is very well fed on vegetables and meat maximum levels are around 30%. This I think is a point which should be considered. Thank you very much.

Summary

For many years the content of linoleic acid has been the only concern when considering the supply of essential fatty acids (EFA) to the developing human. This has led to very unbalanced EFA diets, with extremely high w6/w3 ratios. In the case of parenteral nutrition, several preparations have appeared, some with a proportion of linoleate to linolenate (18:2w6/18:2w3) very high, and some maintaining a theoretically correct proportion of these fatty acids but supplying a large excess of linoleic acid.

We have studied a small group of perinatal infants fed on total parenteral nutrition (TPN) with the latter type of preparation (Intralipid). These infants died during the neonatal period due to major surgical problems, after having received TPN for 4-12 days, and their liver and brain were studied for the fatty acid composition of ethanolamine and choline phosphoglycerides (FPG and CPG). The fatty acid patterns of these two phosphoglycerides were compared to those obtained in controls of the same gestational age. The most striking finding in the liver of the infants receiving TPN was a great decrease in the proportion of 22:6w3 (docosahexaenoic acid) in EPG and CPG. As for the w6 series, arachidonic acid (20:4w6) was decreased in liver CPG, and the content of linoleic acid was increased in both liver phosphoglycerides, indicating a diminished elongation/desaturation of this fatty acid to longer members of the series. In the brain, the only finding was a significant increase of 18:2w6 in CPG, the longer polyunsaturated fatty acids (PUFA) being within normal limits, in CPG as well as in EPG.

In agreement with the well-known enzymatic competition between families of fatty acids, our findings indicate that an excessive supply of linoleate, especially when given intravenously, can be very dangerous to the developing human in altering the w3/w6 proportion of tissue long PUFA. Even if maintaining a correct w6/w3 ratio, a large excess of precursors can lower the proportion of long PUFA by a mechanism of substrate inhibition, especially if preformed long polyunsaturated fatty acids are not simultaneously provided.

Dicussion

Prof Navarro: Thank you very much for your very interesting data and the paper is open for discussion.

Dr Bjerve: I want to congratulate you with a lot of very important data and they will of course be very important when considering how to prepare formulas for the future. However I'm not quite sure I agree with your interpretations of the mechanisms of why, what does it mean. As far as I understood you interpret these data that there must be some sort of inhibition in desaturation elongation. There are several other possible explanations as well. As far as I recall you didn't measure the total pool size on none of the phospholipids so you don't know whether you increased the total pool size or the EPG or the CPG, that's one thing. You could imagine that you drastically increased one type of species. You will presumably have a very large excess of 18:2n-6 present which will then go into the phospholipids and they will compete with the other long chain fatty acids. That doesn't necessarily mean you will have a lesser supply of the long chain arachidonic acid, eicosapentanoic acid for those sides where the phospholipase A2 connected to prostaglandin synthesis for instance is connected, so one should be very cautions using such data to conclude on the mechanism. However I think they are very important as a way to try to estimate what kind of formulas do we need or do we want for the children. Thank you.

Dr Huang: Do you have a measure in DA, the brain weight during the growth, during that period and what's the pool size of the CPG and the EPG during those changes.

Dr Martinez: You mean if I measured the phospholipids. Yes there were no significant changes, in percentage.

Dr Bourre: In fact I have three questions. The first question is related to the total amount. At the beginning of your presentation you say there is a decrease in arachidonic acid and an increase in DHA but in fact due to the increase of all phospholipids during the developing period. Then it could be possible that arachidonic acid is stable and DHA is even more increased. So you don't have any data on the total amount of each individual polyunsaturated fatty acid in terms of quantity. The other point is what about the blood contamination in your samples, because it could be possible that the increase you see in linolenic acid in the TPN treated patients could be due to the blood as the brain only contains trace amounts of linolenic acid and linoleic acid so it is very easy to increase the amount just by very low blood contamination. Could it be possible?

Dr Martinez: I don't think so, not in this proportion. The tissues were very well whashed, then the phospholipids were separated. I don't think small contamination with blood can cause such important changes. And in any case we are comparing tissues which have been studied in the same manner in all the children, in any case there would be blood contamination in all the cases.

Dr Bourre: And the last point, at least for us, is when reducing linolenic acid or increasing linoleic acid in the diet the best index is always an increase in a 22:5n-6, which is virtually drastically increased. So you haven't presented any data of these fatty acids. Did you find some changes?

Dr Martinez: No these fatty acids were not changed, these have been publisheed in full in the paper I just wanted to be brief and to present the more significant changes. There were not important changes either in 22:4 or 22:5 omega 6, not in the liver. There is an important change in the brain during development of the index 22:4 to 22:5 in normal situation. There was no change in the total parentally nourished children and there was no important change of the index in the liver, because in the liver in relation to the other fatty acids these two are quite minor. They are very important in the brain but not in the liver and the changes of these two fatty acids as I say were not significant at all. But I have published all the data in full. Just I wanted to specify over these two and to present the data case by case I think it is important because I have to make three groups for the publication and it is better. Some changes are so subtile that it is better to follow all the age span and not just by group.

Dr Messing: My question is what was the quantity per kilo and per day of intralipid you infuse and what was the proportion of this quantity related to the normal neonates feeding, and last point do you use 10 or 20%?

Dr Martinez: It is 20%, the proportion is 4g/kilo/day increasing from 1 to 4 in the course of 7 days to be slowly and this is the general practice in our hospital.

Dr Messing: Can you correlate the duration of your TPN regimen between 4 and 12 days and the per cent change in comparison with the controls? I mean if your duration is longer have you more important change?

Dr Martinez: We don't know that you know. I have to take the tissues as they come to my hands because this is not the animal experiments; so these were children who died and it was the reason why I could have access to the tissues and other children who survived we could not collect any. We have been studying also the effect, I must tell you it's surely one case but I think it is important in this respect. The effect of a very unbalanced diet orally, not parenterally, but really unbalanced by unbalanced I mean with more than 200 ratio between linoleic and alphalinolenate, and this child was a premature who had been born at about 24 weeks of gestational age, and then was being fed in my hospital with this diet which is very common and this was very mature and could not be recovered, the weight was increasing quite nicely but she had lung complication and died then I could study the brain and the retina of this child, and I must tell you that the retina was about half also about half, this time in quantitative terms because nowadays; I must tell you this is an old work so I did this analysis only qualitative and with a packed column. Now I'm working quantitative and with a capillary column and I must tell you that this docosahexanoic fatty acid in the retina was half exactly the amount it should have in the normal situation compared with a child of the same post-conceptional age, because this child died at more than a month of age which corresponded to about 44 weeks of a full term baby and the docosahexanoic was half, so I think we should be very careful about the supply of omega 3 to the brain. As for the mechanism I agree that I was just suggesting a mechanism, I myself cannot understand why but these are facts and I think that if we are faced with these kind of facts we should change the feeding.

Dr Chairman: Two more questions but if you permit I just want to add a question. Have you some data about the structural modification in the exams you were able to perform and because I want to say when you speak of the dangerous aspect, have you observed some structural change in brain for example in those cases?

Dr Martinez: No, we haven't, we now are planning to do the electro-retinogram in children which is a nice way of doing it in vivo. We have not, I think perhaps there is a period when you cannot change anything microscopically with something more subtle. I judge it is good to be in time of sensing things before they express in a deficiency of a bigger size.

Dr Ghisolfi: For explaining the decrease of the delta 6 desaturase activity perhaps there is another explanation, it is the very severe pathological state of your patient during TPN. What do you think of this hypothesis?

Dr Martinez: Well these children receiving parenteral nutrition were surgical children, I mean they were quite fast, I don't know all children who died are severely ill so I don't know if we can condlude anything form this.

Dr Ghisolfi: But the functions of the liver were not normal in these patients and this can explain the decrease of the delta 6 desaturase activity.

Dr Martinez: You mean the patient receiving TPN?

Dr Ghisolfi: Yes.

Dr Martinez: I don't know, we don't have any data showing this, any liver abnormality you know, it was what kind of death quite fast.

Dr Friedman: Dr Martinez thank you very much for the interesting information. I would just like to ask you were these babies in anabolic or catabolic stage, were they receiving enough calories?

Dr Martinez: Yes, I think so.

Dr Friedman: The weight death was below birth rate?

Dr Martinez: In the moment of death you say? No they were kept in good condition, I mean they were within percentals which are correct for the age.

Dr Friedman: This information is a bit disturbing that there was such a drastic change in biochemistry in such a short time. The problem that I have is that extra-uterine growth is completely different from intra-uterine in all the aspects and we cannot compare it to brain biochemistry in infants who are being fed for example breast milk, there is no comparison; so we really don't know what's the natural cause post-uterine and this is what I have difficulties with.

Dr Martinez: Yes you are right there, I just happen not to have any liver for children fed breast milk, it could be nice. I have even thought to try to correlate the phospholipid fatty acid patterns in a live tissue as erythrocyte membrane to these other tissues to see if I can do some kind of a study of human breast fed milk babies compared to the others, which these are artificial milk which all of them, most all of them are more or less unbalanced.

12

Does cutaneous application of essential fatty acids (EFA) prevent EFA deficiency during total parenteral nutrition in infants

O. GOULET, C. RICOUR

Service de gastroentérologie et nutrition, Hôpital des Enfants Malades, 149 rue de Sèvres, 75730 Paris Cedex 15, France.

Prof. Ghisolfi, Mr Chairman, Kabivitrum team, ladies and gentlemen thank you very much to give me the opportunity to be there. I am going to present some data on cutaneous application of essential fatty acid rich oil. The first part concerns a study performed by us in Paris with Dr Ricour and Dr Bouclet. In the second part I will present some data from the literature. Essential fatty acid deficiency appears within the first day of fat free parenteral nutrition, this was shown by Pallsrud in 1972 and more recently by others authors. Pallerud in 72 showed and increase in eicosatrienoic acid after some day of fat free TPN and a decrease of arachidonic acid. Clinical symptoms in infants are limited and delayed regarding to biological change. Attempts to prevent or to correct EFA deficiency by cutaneous application of EFA rich oil has given conflicting results. We designed this clinical study in infants on TPN in order to evaluate the effect of an EFA rich oil cutaneous application on plasma EFA levels, second to correlate plasma EFA levels to cellular status.

Patients

Patients were separated into two groups according to oil cutaneous application or not. The first group includes 10 patients aged 4 months studied during 24 days of TPN and with oil application. The second group (6 patients) was a same age group with TPN treatment a little bit lower, without any oil application.

Parenteral intakes were the same in both groups, without any intravenous fat emulsion administration. Adequate amounts of trace elements were provided especially for zinc, copper and iron. Caloric intake was 100 kcal per kilo per day in each group. Group 1 received application of œnethera oil on the largest cutaneous surface available using vinyl gloves. Application was performed using .8 ml/kg, three times a day during twenty minutes for twenty days, that provided almost 2 g of EFA per kilo, per day. Œnethera oil is quite a rich oil in EFAs omega 6 and also omega 3 but much lower.

Blood samples were collected on the 1 and 20 in each group of the study. Control patients include 10 infants of same age group but without any gastro-intestinal disease and without any TPN and after an overnight fast. We studied fatty acid contents of plasma phospholipids as well as of erythrocyte phospholipids. After lipid extraction the method used gas chromatography; variance analysis was used to statistical method.

Results

About the skin aspects who were quite dry and a little bit scaly at start in both TPN groups, the skin aspect was improved in group 1 only, but not altered in group 2 without any fat adminstration on skin. Results on plasma phospholipids EFA are given as percentage according to normal control group. They showed between day 1 and day 20, first the same change in both TPN group, either in cutaneous EFA supplemented group or non supplemented TPN group: decrease in omega 6 in each group with an increase in eicosatrienoic acid in durint the same period between day 1 and day 2.

The change in plasma fatty acid composition is almost the same for erythrocytes. For omega 6, decrease in linoleic acid and increase c20:3v-9. The value at the start was a little bit different in the TPN group, with fat adminstration compared to the group without fat administration, but the differences were not significant. While fatty acid change was the same in both TPN groups supplemented or not supplemented with cutaneous oil, we put all together the TPN patient and looked for the change in plasma fatty acids. First about saturated and monounsaturated fatty acids of serum phospholipids, we see that in patient TPN group without cutaneous oil compared to an ormal, control group, palmitic acid was increased as well as palmitoleic acid and oleic acids. Omega 6 fatty acids plasma levels were decreased on day 1 and day 20 in both TPN group, compared to normal control group, that for linoleic acid, dihomogammalinolenic acids and arachidonic acid. Triene/tetraene ratio was increased in both TPN groups on day 1 and increased on day 20, meaning probably that EFA deficiency was more important on day 20.

Conclusions

The first conclusion of our study is that cutaneous application of EFA rich oil did not correct TPN induced EFA deficiency. This study has the previous report showed simultaneously change of plasma and red blood cells fatty acid composition althouth red blood cell change were smaller. Several studies have been reported in the literature concerning the effects of EFA rich oils on EFA deficiency. Preast the first in 1974 has corrected EFA deficiency within 15 days by using low amount of sunflower oil in adults, low amount 2-3 mg/kg/d. Friedman reported in 1976 2 cases of newborns with clinical symptoms of essential fatty acids who were treated with 1 g/kg/d of sunflower oil and within 6 days they observed a clinical correction of skin. They obtained also a correction of platelets aggregation and about EFAs plasma level, they find the following results. Linoleic acid was corrected in one patient but remained low in the other one. About arachidonic acid both patients were corrected for arachidonic acid after 6 days and eicosatrienoic acid decreased in both patients within 6 or 7 days. But in that study the fatty acid pattern observed in the red blood cells phospholipids was less obvious than the pattern seen in plasma.

Hearns in 1978 performed in 6 neonates and 4 infants with different amounts of oil and did not obtain any correction of EFA deficiency. Miller more recently in the American Journal of Clinical Nutrition in 1987, reported the correction of plasma levels after safflower oil application in 5 adults. Miller himself concluded very carefully through lack of data from patients with clinical EFA deficiency. On the other hand he asked to be careful about the low omega 3 content in safflower oil.

Gammalinoleic acid has been used by cutaneous application in EFA deficient rats. The radio-activity in plasma, peripheral muscle, but also in the liver, kidney and adipose tissue remain negligeable after 8-hour application. On the contrary radio-activity was increasing with time in subcutaneous tissue and abdominal muscle of the rats. It can be concluded by underlining the potential importance of the use of gamma-linoleic acid in dermatology as well as in cosmetology. In conclusion to these reported in the literature are controversial concerning correction of EFA deficiency induced by fat free TPN. Second even if the EFA rich oil are used to correct skin lesion we think that another way must be found to provide EFA to tissue by using for example IV intralipid. Thank you very much.

Summary

Essential fatty acid (EFA) deficiency may appear within the first days of fat free total parenteral nutrition (TPN). Attempts to correct EFA deficiency by cutaneous application of EFA rich oil have given conflicting results on plasma EFA levels. In order to evaluate the effect of EFA cutaneous application we performed this study in infants on fat free TPN. 10 infants on TPN were rubbed three times daily for 20 days using œnethera oil (80% EFA).

Total EFA amount provided cutaneously was 1900 mg/kg/d. Plasma and RBC phospholipids were determined on days 1 and 20 in these 10 treated and 6 untreated infants on TPN and compared with those of normal control infants. On day 1, plasma non-essential FA including 20:3 n-9 ($p<.01$) were increased in both TPN groups while 18:2 n-6 and 18:3 n-3 ($p<.001$ and $p<.01$) were decreased. On the 20th day, EFA deficiency has worsened with a decrease in plasma level of 20:4 n-6 ($p<.02$) and a higher than normal triene/tretaene ratio: $3.4 + 1$ and $2.3 + 6$ vs $.1 + 1$ ($p<.02$). As for RBC phospholipids, 16:0 was increased and 18:2 n-6 and 20:3 n-6 were decreased ($p<.05$) on day 1. On day 20, these FA were more abnormal while 20:3 n-9 became significantly increased ($p<.05$). No difference was observed between the TPN groups at any time. These results show that cutaneous application of large amounts of EFA rich oil is unable to prevent or cure TPN EFA deficiency.

Discussion

Dr Adam: In Germany we have some ointments containing linoleic acid, but the fact is that most of this linoleic acid in a trans linoleic acid and we know that big differences exist between cis and trans linoleic acid, but I just want to know whether the ointment you used was cis or trans linoleic acid and whether a difference is reported in the literature, may be it can be referred to this point.

Dr Goulet: Œnethera oil content of linoleic acid is cis.

Chairman: Perhaps I would ask about the differences also if you permit and if Dr Friedman also can answer. You compare your result to Dr Friedman's experience and I was asking if there was also a difference between the patients, because Dr Friedman work on neonates and you work on TPN patients, and my question was they were brought before this experience from a long time on a fat free diet because I was very surprised of the high percentage of the 20:3 omega 9 you showed us at the beginning of the study; so perhaps Dr Friedman may answer and after we come back to the other question.

Dr Friedman: Well it's a difficult problem I think the difference in the patients is that the two that we have treated had cutaneous lesions. It's very possible that with an unction of oil and the absorption it's better than on skin without any lesions. Also skins of premature infants is more permeable and you know it in fact not just to water evaporation but to other pharmacological agents. Thirdly we don't know whether there was some absorption of EFA in your study because we really don't have any information on tissue at our level, it's very possible that the absorption even if a minimal absorption is actually even not stored in tissue, but converted immediately to prostaglandins through any other eicosanoids, so we really don't know from this study whether there is absorption, what degree of absorption and what the EFAs are doing, whether they are stored as EFAs or converted immediately to other products. That's basically what I have to answer.

Chairman: Thank you very much. Other questions?

Dr Bourre: I agree with you that in most of the patients you should probably use intralipid and cutaneous application, but there are some patient groups where there is really a problem of applying or giving them enough calories and that's the extremely small low birth infant where you want to give about 120 k/cal per kilogram and that might prove difficult in some cases and even if you are using intralipid because of the delaterous effect. So I think we should explore the possibility of cutaneous application until we really know what's going on and my question to you is in line with Dr Friedman how do you really know that your fatty acid is absorbed, to your supplying 2g of EFA per day divided in three doses in oil containing 80% of EFA. How much would you say resides within the vinyl gloves, how large a part of the body is covered with your oil, do you only rub it on the stomach, on the back, on the arms, I think the absorption problem is a major one when your trying to evaluate these different studies.

Dr Goulet: To answer your question about the measurement of what remains as fat on the gloves for example we did not perform any measurements. Second, the largest part of the body was with application. We don't know and we cannot know what part of the fatty acid was really absorbed or transformed on the subcutaneous parts. What we know that no plasma level as well as erythrocyte level change during the study. I come back very quickly about Dr Friedman comments and I think that permeability is probably the most important point to explain the difference in the different studies, because you cannot imagine that it is dose dependent because some study expose results with very low dose in adults 2-3 mg/kg/d and in infants much more important doses. It's not the quality of the oil because we did not correct by using an oil with a very high level of EFA, more than 80% and in safflower oil for example or sunflower oil, EFA content is less. I think it's a question of permeability, a question of real essential fatty status. In Dr Friedman's patients the patient has real EFA deficiency with clinical symptoms; our patients did not have any symptoms of EFA deficiency as well as the patient of Miller. I think may be the degree or real EFA deficiency can play a role and the third is may be but I don't know if it's real a metabolic state can be different between infants, neonates, premature infants and adult patients.

Dr Bourre: I just would like to come back to the important comment raised by Dr Adam concerning the trans isomer because indeed in some commercial oils huge amounts of trans isomer are found. When feeding rats up to 20% of the linolenic acid for instance sometimes is in the trans form. So if feeding rats for instance with trans isomers of linolenic acid, then it is elongated and desaturated and incorporated into the membrane including the brain which means these fatty acids are totally not physiological and they can change their membrane function and then the function of the cells. So one has to take into the occurrence of trans isomer, you can change everything due to the occurrence of this trans isomer.

Dr Bivins: Has anyone administered EFAs subcutaneously, provided for depot storage in these very small neonates rather than trying to get the oil to pass the cutaneous barrier.

Dr Goulet: I have no answer, may be somebody has an answer, I don't know.

Dr Cunnane: I was curious about the fatty acid data from the plasma and I may have misinterpreted it so perhaps you can explain it because you had a substantial decrease in linoleic acid, arachidonic acid, 20:3 omega 6 and then you showed the 18:1, 16:0 values and so on and they were essentially normal. So what was accounting for the big difference, something must have gone up proportionally if the EFAs had gone down as much as you showed. What was this quantitative data, I didn't quite understand.

Dr Goulet: It may be due to a small number of patients. The monounsaturated and saturated fatty acids were increased; it's true, at the start as well as after 20 days of oil application the saturated and monounsaturated fatty acids 18:0 were increased in both TPN groups and the increase was a little bit higher after 20 days and the level was lower in non-treated patient group, in control group of normal patient.

Dr Hansen: You said your patients has dry skin and I would like to know what about the humidity, because high humidity will decrease the EFA deficiency symtoms, so you can have EFA deficient patients without seeing any clinical symptoms if the humidity is high. The second question have you measured water loss of the skin of these patients.

Dr Goulet: The first question, all the patients were infants, mean age 4 months and no patient were in incubator and the humidity of the atmosphere was the same for all and I hope not too humid and about your second question, we did not measure the water losses of the patient.

Chairman: Thank you Olivier and we have now the pause. Thank you very much.

13

How to appreciate the adequacy supply of essential fatty acid during total parenteral nutrition in clinical practice

J. GHISOLFI

Médecine infantile D, CHR Purpan, 31059 Toulouse Cedex

One of the main actual concerns, when using total parenteral nutrition in human clinical practice, is the appreciation of the adequacy of emulsion administration, particularly in relation to essential fatty acids (EFA). This problem is difficult to approach because of the complexity of essential fatty acid metabolism during total parenteral nutrition TPN and of the inaccessibility of most tissues, in clinical practice, particularly in children.

All our protocols were performed in infants aged from one to four months, receiving total parenteral nutrition for more than one month, indicated because of various digestive diseases. Linoleic acid supply was only in the form of intralipid 20%. During the protocol periods, the infants were in stable clinical and metabolic conditions, had a normal growth rate of 20-32 g/day. All the results obtained, after at least one month of total parenteral nutrition, were compared to those noted in the same infants prior to the study and to those of healthy controls of the same age. Concerning methods, gas chromatography was used for fatty acid analysis in blood and tissues and radio-immunoassay dosages for prostaglandin measurements.

First of all, fatty acid composition of total serum lipids or of serum phospholipids does not reflect essential fatty acid status during total parenteral nutrition. Whatever the levels of linoleic acid supplies, representing about 2.5, 3.5 and 5% of total calories, we never noted, compared to the results observed before the total parenteral nutrition period, and to healthy controls, a normalization of fatty acid profiles. After at least one month of TPN, we always had lower levels of linoleic and arachidonic acids, higher levels of palmitic, oleic, eicosatriensoic acids and of the triene-tetraene ratio. Fatty acid distribution in plasma phospholipid fractions cannot express essential fatty acid status during total parenteral nutrition either. For instance, with 350 mg/kg/day of linoleic acid supply, which represents about 3.5% of total calories, a dose usually considered as sufficient to avoid linoleic acid deficiency, we never obtained after one month a normalisation of linoleic, and eicosatrienoic and of the triene-tetraene ratio, in infants with EFA deficiency status.

Total fatty acid composition of the serum or fatty acid composition of plasma phospholipids are more affected by total parenteral metabolic conditions than by the levels of linoleic acid supplies. These dosages cannot be used to appreciate the adequacy of fat-emulsion administration.

Because of their accessibility, red blood cells or platelets are often studied. After at least one month of fat emulsion administration, a period which is longer than the fatty acid turn over in erythrocytes, we noted, compared to healthy controls receiving the same linoleic acid supply orally, a normalization of the fatty acid distribution, particularly of n-6 fatty acids. Results concerning n-3 fatty acids, particularly long chain n-3 fatty acid have been obtained by other authors showing that erythrocyte fatty acid composition is linked to variations of n-3 fatty acids in the diet. Platelet dosages are not often used, particularly in infants, because of the great quantity of blood which require these measurements but give the same results.

It is possible to obtain another tissue easily, that is cheek cells, collected by having the subjects rinse the mouth with water, or, in infants, by scraping the cheek with a spoon. It has been shown, in adults, that the phospholipid fatty acid composition of human cheek cell reflects dietary lipid status. We also noted that there was, in infants, a correlation between linoleic acid percentage in phospholipid cheek cells and linoleic acid supplies. We also found in orally fed infants, a correlation for both linoleic and arachidonic acid percentages between on the one hand plasma and cheek cell phospholipids, on the other hand, erythrocyte and cheek cell phospholipids. We think that cheek cell phospholipids may represent a good way to study the adequacy of linoleic acid supplies from fat emulsion.

But erythrocyte, platelets, or cheek cells are very particular tissues. Red cell, platelet or check cell phospholipid fatty acid composition probably returns to normal more rapidly than other tissue composition it is well known that fatty acid distribution is different in membranes in function of organs, and for a given tissue is different for each phospholipid. These changes in levels of dietary lipids affected differently the fatty acid composition of membrane phospholipids and therefore modified the properties of the membranes. Tissues respond differently when varying dietary fat and certainly also when varying fat emulsion administration. Analysing only one or two tissues, as erythrocytes, platelets, or cheek, cells is probably not sufficient to appreciate the adequacy of fat emulsion administration. So, it is certainly important to see the effects of fat emulsion administration on various membrane tissues, during total parenteral nutrition. These effects have been studied in animals, or in humans on post morten examination, and given interesting results. However it would be of great interest to obtain data in vivo to adapt fat emulsion administration. For ethical reasons, these dosages are most often not possible to realize.

We have had the opportunity to obtain adipose tissue during the course of an abdominal surgical operation, realized in infants treated by TPN for more than one month. We analyzed the fatty acid composition of adipocyte membrane phospholipids and triglycerides. Compared to healthy controls receiving two times more of linoleic acid supplies orally, no significant difference for both essential or non essential fatty acids in membrane phospholipids was noted. But in another study, we observed in orally fed infants receiving from 250 to 2 000 mg/kg/24 h of linoleic acid supply that the amount of linoleic acid in the diet modulated the percentage of n-6 fatty acid in adipose membrane phospholipids. We did not have data concerning n-3 acids using great variations of C18:3 n-3 supplies. In adipocyte triglycerides, we noted that after one month of TPN, compared to healthy controls of the same age, receiving identical EFA supplies, that the percentage of linoleic acid was significantly lower in TPN infants. We did not observe any significantly change of others fatty acid particularly of n-6 and n-3 families. This decrease in linoleic acid percentage seem to be linked to TPN metabolic conditions. In orally fed infants receiving from 250 to 2 000 mg/kg/24 h of C18:2 n-6, the quantity of each n—6 fatty acid stored in triglycerides is linked to the importance of linoleic acid supply.

It would be interesting to have data for other tissues in humans in vivo during TPN. The results presented during this workshop by Prof. Friedman and Dr M. Martinez show that each tissue composition rapidly and considerably varies during TPN. It has only recently been appreciated that the effects of EFA deprivation on the phospholipid composition of different tissues are quite diverse. In linoleic acid deficient rats, it is observed in liver, kidney and heart phospholipids a decrease of linoleic and arachidonic acid except in phosphotidyl ethanolamine of the heart where it is noted a paradoxical increase of arachidonic acid.

To really appreciate the adequacy of fat emulsion administration during TPN, it would be necessary to have data concerning not only one or two tissues, but almost each tissue, which is evidently impossible to propose in clinical practice.

As variations in fatty acid membrane composition directly affect the properties of the membrane, an interesting approach to study the effect of IV fat emulsion administration is certainly to look at some specific functions which are known to be directly linked to fatty acid membrane composition, as electroretinogram or electrophysiological functions. Infortunately I have no results to present and in my knowledge, no data are known in human TPN conditions. It is certainly an important way to examine in the future.

Another way to study essential fatty acid status is to evaluate prostaglandin urinary excretion. There is a close relationship between dietary fats and prostaglandin urinary excretion. As other authors, we noted this correlation. We observed that PGE_1, PGE_2 and PGF_2 alpha urinary excretion was normalized in TPN infants by 350 or 550 mg/kg/day of linoleic acid supplies, but not by 250 mg/kg/day which represents however 2.5% of total calories. We did not find any correlation between fatty acid distribution, particularly arachidonic acid percentage, in plasma or erythrocyte phospholipids and prostaglandin urinary excretion. It would appear that prostaglandin urinary more represents linoleic acid supplies from fat emulsion than fatty acid content in tissues. It is not linked to prostaglandin precursor available in membranes, mainly arachidonic acid. It is probable that measurement of urinary prostaglandin excretion is not a reliable index of renal or other tissue prostaglandin synthesis, and therefore of EFA status.

From these data, how can we appreciate the adequacy of a fat emulsion during TPN in clinical practice?

• *And first, how can appreciate the minimum or optimum linoleic acid requirement in patients during TPN?* Administration of only 1 to 2% of calories in the form of linoleic acid will support normal growth and development and prevent clinical appearance of essential fatty acid deficiency. But the clinical criteria are certainly not sufficient. We saw that to study fatty acid composition of total serum lipids or plasma phospholipids is not adequate. In the same way, to determine the minimum amount of linoleic acid in order to maintain the classical ratio triene-tetraene below 0.2 in different tissues does not permit the detection of marginal linoleic acid deficiency. It is probably necessary to compare several data. From our results concerning fatty acid dosages in erythrocytes, cheek cells and adipose tissue, and prostaglandin urinary measurements, 250 mg/kg/day seem to be insufficient and 350 mg/kg/day, (3.5% of total calories) sufficient. But is it really enough to maintain optimal membrane functions and tissue prostaglandin biosynthesis? It is impossible to reply. The definition of an essential fatty acid inadequate status is still arbitrary and indistinct.

• *Second question, do these emulsions, despite their relatively high linoleic acid content, permit normal prostaglandin synthesis?* Several studies showed, in infants, as well as in adults, that high levels of linoleic acid supplies during TPN can have an inhibitory effect on n-6 fatty acid metabolism and prostaglandin synthesis. However, very often, intravenous linoleic acid from fat emulsion usually administered represents more than 10% of calories during TPN in adults and, apparently these patients have no problem. On the contrary, when comparing TPN infants and healthy controls, receiving the same linoleic acid supply, we noted, both in erythrocytes and cheek cell phospholipids, lower level of linoleic acid and higher level of gamma linolenic, dihomogamma linolenic and arachidonic acids. With very high linoleic acid intake, in children receiving a constant rate enteral nutrition, which brings more than 2 000 mg/kg/day of linoleic acis, we never noted a decrease of the higher homologues of linoleic acid, in erythrocyte, adipocyte or cheek cell phospholipids. However Prof Friedman and Dr M. Martinez during this workshop showed that during TPN delta 6 desaturase could be insufficient, leading to an accumulation of linoleic acid in all tissues, and a decrease of prostaglandin urinary excretion. Certainly IV fat emulsion administration has to be made with caution when a pathologic state can induce a decrease of desaturase activities. This problem remains to debate and rise the question of the interest of oil-rich in gamma linolenic acid.

• *Another question is: are long-chain polyunsaturated fatty acids of interest, particularly in infants during TPN?* It is probably easy to reply using erythrocyte and cheek cell phospholipid dosages. Studies showed that these long-chain fatty acids are higher in these phospholipid fractions in human milk fed infants than in artificially fed infants. We noted that during total parenteral nutrition in infants, erythrocyte and cheek cell phospholipids contain less of the 20 to 22 carbon polyunsaturated fatty acids than do human milk infants. Perhaps, it is important, for paediatric practice to consider that fat emulsion has to contain n-3 or n-6 long chain polyunsaturated fatty acids as in human milk, but it is now impossible to propose a response based on objective data.

To conclude the classical biochemical parameters do not clearly permit to define the optimal supply of fat emulsion during total parenteral nutrition, for normal physiological function. Further studies are needed including, as several reports in this meeting have show, cell capacity for prostaglandin synthesis, specific cell function such as platelet aggregation but also the study of tissue membrane properties.

Discussion

Prof Navarro: Thank you Jacques, and now the paper is open for discussion.

Prof Adam: I was very impressed by your data and above all by the difference you found in the plasma and in the tissues which you investigated. You did note an adequate increase of linoleic acid in spite of supply of about 2.1 gr, if I calculated right with your data. My question is whether the linoleic acid content of these tissues may be reduced by the illness of patient and may be a consequence of the situation of the patient or should be whether we have any parameter which gives us some information about the need for linoleic acid in a special patient. I think there is not a uniform need for linoleic acid but it is very individual depending on the situation.

Prof Ghisolfi: I agree completely with your remarks. It is impossible to define for a population an optimal supply because optimal supply is only an individual parameter. To reply to the second question I had not enough time to explain exactly our methodology but our TPN conditions were only in infants without severe digestive diseases and with a good growth which was about 20-32 gr/day. They were in a good metabolic, good nutritional condition. I don't think this factor can act.

Dr Cunnane: In TPN there must be a totally different lipoprotein profile which is going to be present in the blood and presumably the availability of linoleic acid to the peripheral tissues in the lipoprotein lipase is not going to be active in the same way. Is there anybody who has any information on this and particularly perhaps a comparison between similar clinical conditions if it's possible, enteral and parenteral nutrition.

Prof Ghisolfi: I agree completely with you, it's difficult to compare different conditions.

Dr Cunnane: Is there anything known about the lipoprotein distribution or the composition in such infants under these sort of studies?

Prof Ghisolfi: I cannot reply.

Dr Koletzko: These are really very elegant studies that you have presented. You raised the point that the concentration of long chain polyunsaturated fatty acids may depend on the dose of intralipid given. What is your intralipid dose.

Prof Ghisolfi: We used about 2 gram per kilogram per day.

Dr Koletzko: The second question is, you showed that this impressive difference between different compartments plasma, phospholipids and so forth. Did you analyse the plasma phospholipids during lipid infusion?

Prof Ghisolfi: No, never, we obtained the samples after 24 hours without lipid infusion, during TPN only with glucose and amino acid infusion.

Chairman: About the interest of your cheek cell study, I observed there was a big difference concerning arachidonic acid. Do you think, between erythrocyte and cheek cells, there is something different about the explanation of the repartition of the fatty acids or there is only the practical aspect of taking the cheek cells that interest you.

Prof Ghisolfi: I cannot reply today to this important question but we are studying this problem, but I cannot reply now exactly.

Prof Friedman: I would like to comment on the last question that you asked. One of the differences between cheek cells and the red blood cells is that the half life of cheek. I believe is going to be 72 hours or 96 hours. So I think the difference in the distribution of cell membrane phospholipid may be different in red blood cells which has 120 days or 100 in the newborns.

Dr Adam: Again I should like to come back to the data you gave for arachidonic acid and you found parenteral nutrition no decrease of arachidonic acid compared to the controls but oral nutrition a decrease from 10-12% of arachidonic acid. You showed us that parenteral nutrition increased urinary prostaglandins and you speculated that the relation between arachidonic acid and prostaglandin formation might be different in parenteral nutrition and oral nutrition and I should like that you can comment on that.

Prof Ghisolfi: I don't say that prostaglandin biosynthesis is different in function of orally or total parenteral conditions but what I want to say that we did not find any correlation between fatty acid content in tissues and prostaglandin urinary excretion. This point is probably very important. Prostaglandin urinary excretion is not linked to kidney fatty acid content.

14

Omega-3 essential fatty acid deficiency and artificial nutrition

K.S. BJERVE

Department of clinical chemistry, Regional Hospital, University of Trondheim, N 7006 Trondheim, Norway

Mr Chairman, Prof Ghisolfi, first I would like to thank you all for the opportunity to come here to speak to you in Toulouse. It has been a very agreeable meeting and I am certainly happy to be able to present some of the results we have to you. What I am going to talk about, is some patients we have been able to study having a very low intake of omega 3 fatty acids and a normal or low normal intake of omega 6 fatty acids. These patients have all been fed by enteral tube feeding from 2 to 12 years of time this is a summary of these patients, some of the patients have received an oral speciality called where the fat source is a mixture of cornoil, milk fat. Four of the patients have received .02% of the calories as omega 3s, .5 to .6% as omega 6. One patient received a same type of diet, this was a 90 year old lady, three patients received the same diet but prepared slightly differently receiving .05 to .09% of calories from omega 3 and 1.3 up to 2.8% from omega 6. I will also present some results from one patient, a girl receiving a diet where the major fat source was sunflower seed oil and also some fat from MCT. We are studying some other /patients presently, one of them is an old lady where nearly 4% of the calories comes from omega 6, there is low amount from omega 3, she is presently receiving pure eicosapentanoic acid ethyl ester.

Considering a map of Europe Norway. The patients I'm going to describe live on the western coast of Norway.

This is a picture of the forearm of a 90 year old lady. She had received a special diet for two years and had received about 0.02% of calories from omega 3, 0.6% of calories from omega 6 fatty acids. This is how she looked, her skin was covered with these scaly flakes. We started to give her pure alphalinolenic acid and this is her forearm 6 days later. This is the effect of supply of a very small amount of pure alphalinolenic acid for a rather short time. A 26 year old man had received total enteral, artificial nutrition for 12 years, a little more than 12 years. He had this dermatitis covering his whole face. We started giving him pure alphalinolenic acid and he received this alphalinolenic acid two weeks using .1 ml per day followed by two other weeks with half .5 ml per day. This is after four weeks and I hope you agree that his forehead is getting better. When we changed to pure, partly pure fishoil containing approximately 50% omega 3 fatty acids, his skin doesn't contain this dermatitis any longer.

Two of the patients had a folliculitis, the scalp was covered by infections and after 10 days of pure alphalinolenic acid all the infection in the scalp had disappeared. There was still quite a lot of seborrhae which eventually also disappeared when we started to give the purified fishoil preparation.

Another patient, a 30 year old woman received oral tube feeding for 10 years, she had had this very usual pressure it had remained unchanged for one and a half year and it looks just like any other pressure ulcer. We started to give her alphalinolenic acid and within 10 days the nurses reported changes in the ulcer. Four weeks later, the original edges of the ulcer is out and one and a half months after this the ulcer had completely closed. No other things were done except supply this lady with omega 3 fatty acids, her treatment were the same as she had before.

Now let us consider the mean fatty acid changes in erythrocytes before supplementation of the three patients we have looked at, the eicosapentanoic acid, arachidonic acid, total omega 6 fatty acids. You can see the total omega 3 fatty acids values are low compared with the control values for the omega 3s, while the values for omega 6 are normal. When we give .1 ml of alphalinolenic acid for 14 days all omega 3 and omega 6 fatty acids fell quite drastically and we don't know why. We don't think it's an artifact. We have checked it in the ways we were able to by running normals at the same time, checking, reanalysing we get the same results. We cannot explain it. Increasing 2.5 ml per day of alphalinolenic acid, we come back to normal, or not normal, but the initial values, going back changing to the oil .5 ml per day, we now start to see a normalization of the values and we also see quite a drastic increase of the omega 6 values.

In these three patients we also quantitate fatty acids in Lymphocytes. Before suppling omega 3s, we had a mean percentage of 37 and after 4 weeks of alphalinolenic acid this had increased to 58% increasing further to 70% after another four weeks of the purified fishoil. This is the way the white blood cells reacts to mutagens in these patients. This column tells us how the cells incorporate when not stimulated, it's a background value. The upper line shows the stimulation value before starting supplement with omega 3 fatty acids. You can see using concanavaline A we have a stimulated incorporation of nearly 60 000 into the white cells. This is drastically reduced after four weeks of alphalinolenic acid supplementation and even further reduced when you change to the partially purified fishoil. You see about the same picture also when you use pokeweed mutagen as a stimulant.

I'm now going to show you some data from a seven year old girl, she had received per oral tube nutrition from the age of three. The last three years she had received a preparation containing 16% of calories from omega 6 fatty acids and .07% from omega 3 fatty acids. This is her fatty acid values in plasma, total plasma lipids in March 86 before we started supplement and the reason for my showing it is to show you she initially had a very low amount of eicosapentanoic acid, docosapentanoic and docosahexanoic acid. You can see her concentration of omega 6 fatty acids were increased above so called normal or reference range. Low omega 3 high omega 6 and you can see when we started supplement, first with a combination with linseed oil and a small dose of cod liver oil and secondly with just cod liver oil we get the expected increase in the omega 3s. This is just to show you low omega 3 which increases when you supplement this girl as we should expect. We had a very good weight measurement of this girl. She had not changed her weight for the last one and a half year and she was also very low in weight, about 10 kilos at the time we started to study her. At this point we gave her 1 ml of linseed oil and .2 ml of cod liver oil per day, and she increases her weight near 0.5 kg per month. At this time point, we changed to 7.5 ml of ordinary cod liver oil and there is a slight further increase in the rate of weight gain, but about .64 kilograms per month. At this time, the nurses said she is growing out of her clothes and we realised we didn't know how long this girl was, we measured her and again five months later and she had increased 5 cm in length, so not only did she gain weight she also started to grow in length. These curves only show the extremely low intake of alphalinolenic acid which increases when we change to supplement linseed oil and here the long chain omega 3 when we go to the cod liver oil supplement. Just to show you the high intake of omega 6 fatty acids throughout and this is only to show you the caloric intake. But the point is we started to increase weight when we supplied rather small amounts of omega 3 fatty acids.

What is the biochemical basis of n–3 essentiality and this is speculation, I know. But if we try to summarize the results we have seen in a total of 13 patients now, as the observed skin symptoms in our patients. They are clearly different from those that are seen in omega 6 fatty acid deficiency. We might speculate whether the omega 3 fatty acids has specific functions in cell growth and we might speculate whether they have specific function in immunological incompetent cells. Some of these things are supported by other results from in vitro cell culture results as well.

If we try to use our data to calculate a dietary requirement, one can of course not do that very accurate from a total of 9 patients. But if we say there is a linear relationship between intake and observed concentration of omega 3 fatty acids, we have tried to say what do we need per day to reach the lower normal limit of omega 3 fatty acids in plasma lipids. If we do that we can calculate that need about 290 to 390 mg/day in adults, which is .2 to .3 of calories, then we will have omega 3 values in plasma lipids which is on the lower reference range in normals and if we want to be in the middle on the normal reference range we have to increase this to about 900 mg/day or about 1% of calories. If we do the same type of estimation for the long chain omega 3 fatty acids, we can estimate an intake of 100 or 200 mg/day or .1 to .2% of calories, that will result in a low normal value of omega 3 fatty acods in plasma lipids. If we want to be in the middle of the normal reference range in plasma lipids, we need to have an intake of about 350-400 mg/day which is approximately 4% of total calories. Thank you.

Summary

It is well documented that linoleic acid is an essential fatty acid in man. Alpha-linolenic acid and other n–3 fatty acids are essential in several animal species, although they have not previously been considered essential in man. Through a systematic search for patients fed diets supplying 0.02%-0.09% of total calories from n–3 fatty acids, 8 adults and one child with n–3 fatty acid deficiency have been found. These patients had an intake of n–6 fatty acids ranging from 0.5% to 16.2% of total calories.

In four patients, skin atrophy with a dandruff-like, scaly dermatitis disappeared upon supplementation with both n–3 and n–6 acids. This supplement increased n–3 acids in plasma and erythrocyte lipids, while n–6 acids fell or remained constant. In one 90 year-old woman, similar skin changes started to disappear after 5 days supplement with 0.1 ml pure ethyl linolenate daily. This increased erythrocyte content of both 22:6n–3 and total n–6 fatty acids, while 18:3n–3 and 20:5n–3 remained low.

One 7-year-old girl had been fed by gastric tube since the age of three. Her weight (10.3 kg) had not changed the last 15 months. She was supplemented with 0.9 ml of linseed oil and 0.1 ml of cod-liver oil daily. This induced a weight gain which averaged 0.43 kg/month. Changing the supplement to 7.5 ml of cod liver oil daily increased the weight gain to 0.64 kg/month, and gave an average growth of 1 cm/month.

Three adults aged 27 to 40 years were followed simultaneously. All three showed skin atrophy and a dandruff-like dermatitis. Two of them had an extensive hemorrhagic folliculitis of the scalp, and one an extensive, hemorrhagic dermatitis of the face. They were supplemented with increasing doses of pure ethyl linolenate, followed by increasing doses of a highly purified fish oil (EPA-oil). Skin changes started to normalize within 10 days after supplementing with 0.1 ml of ethyl linolenate daily. Ethyl linolenate reduced the mitogenic response of isolated lymphocytes towards Concanavalin A and Pokeweed mitogen significantly, and EPA-oil reduced the response towards Concanavalin A even further; simultaneously, CD2 positive T-lymphocytes increased significantly from 37% to 70% of mononuclear cells. No significant changes were observed in the urinary output of PGI2-M, bleeding time or peripheral nerve conductivity, and there was no change in the maximal platelet capacity for thromboxane biosynthesis.

The patients represent the first 8 adults and the second child described having n–3 fatty acid deficiency. The results indicate that n–3 fatty acids are essential for normal growth and cell function in man in a similar way as they are essential in several animal species. The symptoms of n–3 fatty acid deficiency are different from those seen in n–6 fatty acid deficiency. The results indicate that n–3 fatty acid deficiency impairs the incorporation of essential n–6 acids into cell membranes. Assuming linear relationship between dietary intake and the measured concentrations of n–3 acids in plasma and erythrocyte lipids, the intake of 18:3n–3 required to give mid-normal plasma and erythrocyte lipid concentrations of n–3 acids has been calculated to 800-1 100 mg/day. The corresponding intake of very long chain n–3 fatty acids was calculated to 300 mg-400 mg daily. The results indicate that dietary requirements of n–3 as well as of n–6 acids should be stated as mg or g per day.

Discussion

Prof Navarro: Thank you very much for a very interesting paper and original data and the paper is open for discussion.

Dr Bourre: Do you have some histological data showing what about the skin because as far as I know only linoleic acid is involved in glycosyl ceramide which are involved in the tie junction in the cells. So you probably have a totally different mechanism to suggest. So can you tell where is the defects in the cells, microsomes and the plasmic reticulum of mitochondria, the cell membranes for instance.

Dr Bjerve: To you first point we don't have microscopic exams of the skin we don't have biopsis. To your second point we don't know anything about the mechanism we can only speculate. I'm pretty sure it's not, the essentiality of omega 3s is not that they make a specific type of protein binding or ceramide binding in the skin as you know is the case for the linoleic acid but I think the skin symptoms we have seen are purely coincidental, they are probably a result of a combination of some setting these patients are in and their low omega 3 fatty acid intake and it's a combination not only the omega 3 fatty acid intake but also some other precipitated effect that determines whether these patients will have skin lesions or not. My best guess at the present is that the skin symptoms we see is not specifically related to omega 3 fatty acid function in the skin, but might be more likely an indication of some other cell system for instance white blood cells, macrophages changing their function precipitating another type of reaction towards inflammatory stimuli, things like that.

Dr Koletzko: Christian, I think that is extremely interesting data that you present and they really give a lot of food for thought, as you know I do not completely agree with your conclusions. We have discussed that previously but I can see that we are getting closer and closer in our ideas, I do not want to repeat this discussion, everybody who is interested can read it in American Journal of Clinical Nutrition last year, part of the discussion was published and it is continued in this June's issue. The questions that I wanted to raise, number 1, is, I am very glad that you are not talking anymore about alphalinolenic acid deficiency but you are now more referring to the sum of omega 3 fatty acids or the long chain metabolites. The first question is, do you think that there is a specific requirement for alphalinolenic acid rather than for omega 3 fatty acid. The second question I have, you have shown this increase in weight in the 7 year old girl, do you think that the prior increase of energy intake could have had a delayed effect such as you sometimes see in malnourished patients where it may take quite a while after giving an increase in the diet as we can sometimes see for example is anorectic patients before you see a weight gain. The third question refers to the interaction, you have shown this extremely interesting data on the interaction between omega 3 and omega 6 fatty acids, do you have any speculation on what might have happened there?

Dr Bjerve: If I start on commenting on the caloric intake in this girl, that's of course a very important question. The increase when we added this alphalinolenic acid as linseed oil and a small dose of cod liver oil, that increased her intake of calories from 750-755 calories per day so it's a very small increase in intake and of course we cannot totally exclude that it's a delayed response but it's a little bit too delayed so I don't believe it. The other thing is to maintain a reasonable weight gain and not to get fat we are now back to 550 k/cal/day in this young girl. So we are even below the initial level before we started to have a fairly normal gain of weight, these data haven't been published but that's what has really happened, which again speaks against its being a pure caloric phenomena. But again it's only one patient, you have to keep that in mind it's only one patient.

Dr Koletzko: May I just ask the other two questions again. Do you think there's a specific requirement for alphalinolenic acid? Do you have a speculation of omega 3 omega 6 interaction ?

Dr Bjerve: Well I hoped you had forgotten! I don't know whether there is any specific requirement for alphalinolenic acid, we don't have any data for it. It seems to work, we have used pure alphalinolenic acid, we have used a rather pure oil, we cannot say one is qualitatively different from the other, we cannot say that. I do not have any explanation why we see this concommitant increase in omega 6 within the cell.

Dr Cunnane: I congratulate you on a splendid piece of work and something that's really difficult I'm sure to do, specially in the logistical situation that you're in. I think that your explanation for the repair of the skin symptoms of the folliculitis is probably on track when you refer to the immune system because alphalinolenic acid has a known bacteriacidal, fungacidal, virusidal effect and I think that is probably connected to, not necessarily as you say to a repair of skin tissue itself. The other point that I wanted to make is I think that the issue of alphalinolenic acid oxidation is probably relevant to the changes in the omega 6s that your seeing in the erythrocytes or was it plasma on the single slide which you didn't discuss a lot but the linoleic acid levels in fact re-elevated after the alphalinolenic acid and I think that this in fact suggests a reduced requirement to use linoleic acid for oxidation and in fact to provide some alpha-linolenic for oxidation, it's pure speculation but is might account for the change that you see.

Dr Bjerve: Yes we have discussed that as a major possibility in the paper, I agree with you.

Dr Huang: In those patients you have shown neurological symptoms?

Dr Bjerve: They had major neurological symptoms all of them, because that was their primary disease, they had large brain damages either from anaesthesia, haemorrhages, from enzymatic inherited enzymatic deficiencies, so because of the primary disease we were not able to examine their SNC functions.

Dr Huang: Is there any improvement after treatment?

Dr Bjerve: No, we wouldn't even expect it. What we did was we looked for changes in the EEGs which we had the possibility to do there are none. They are extremely pathological beforehand and remain so afterwards. There are no differences in peripheral nerve productivity that's the only thing we have.

Dr Adam: I heard that you have some old ladies in your patients and we have done some studies on the n–3 metabolism in old persons and we found some differences on delta 6 desaturase and so I should like to ask you whether you found any special effect of your diet in those old people and whether you think there is other minimal requirement for n–3 fatty acid in older people.

Dr Bjerve: I would not like to comment on that on the basis of these very very few patients which obviously are sick in a lot of ways. We are at present doing a large series of studies in fact including nearly 500 individuals, a little more than 500 individuals of the age of 40 and up to 70 and when we are ready with that we might probably be able to say something about it, but I don't think I will be able to comment from these few patients.

Chairman: Thank you very much.

15

New fatty acids in the emulsions of the nineties. Possibilities and limitations

C.M.H. CARNEHEIM, C. LARSSON-BACCKSTRÖM, L. EKMAN

Kabivitrun Nutrition AB, S-11287 Stockholm, Sweden

The safety and efficacy of present fat emulsions is well documented. Adult patients subjected to long term lipid emulsion treatment have not developed an essential fatty acid syndrome. This indicates that the present emulsion serves as an energy source and as a source of essential fatty acids. Still there are several possibilities to further improve the lipid emulsion, such as:
— optimising the fatty acid pattern;
— improving the emulsifying system;
— improving the stability in all-in-one mixtures;
— making the emulsion more chylomicron-like.

All of the listed points will increase the efficacy, the convenience or both. Regulatory authorities regard a lipid emulsion as comparable with a drug if administered intravenously. This implies that a new lipid emulsion for intravenous use should have an efficacy beyond the already established emulsions. Moreover the safety/efficacy ratio will be carefully scrutinized.

In this review we will only focus on the first point, namely optimising the fatty acid pattern, and thereby adapting the emulsion to specific clinical needs.

Gamma-linolenic acid

Several symptoms in pathophysiologic conditions such as prematures, hepatic cirrhosis, cystic fibrosis, inflammatory bowel diseases, ulcerative colitis, diabetes mellitus and dermatological diseases have been correlated with a low plasma concentration of gamma-linolenic acid. However, by the supplementation of gamma-linolenic acid it may be possible in the newborn/premature or in patients suffering from inflammatory bowel diseases to prove a clinical effect of the fatty acids. Friedman and Frolich [1] have demonstrated that children treated with Intralipid® showed a decrease in PGE-M concentration (*figure 1*). A decrease in PGE-M concentration

Essential fatty acids

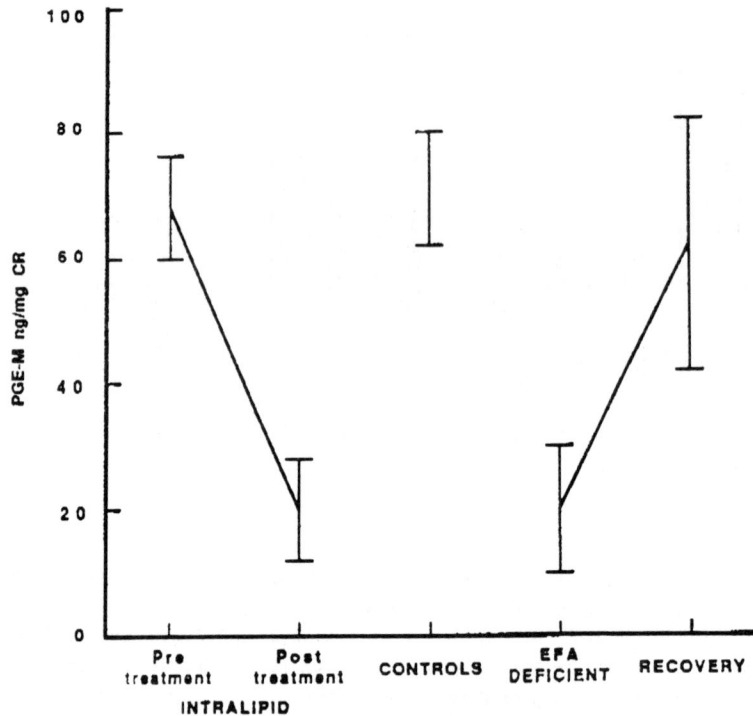

Figure 1. Adapted from [1].

indicates either a decrease in delta-6-desaturase activity or low concentrations of gamma-linolenic acid, as PGE-M is one of the products in the metabolism of w6 fatty acids. The PGE-M concentration after Intralipid® treatment was in the same order as in children with EFA-deficiency. It is possible from this study to conclude that a supplementation of gamma-linolenic acid may improve the emulsion when given to premature or newborn children. However, it has to be pointed out that this effect may as well be regulated by a far more complex mechanism involving the balance between the w3 and w6 fatty acids.

ω3-fatty acids

The balance between the ω3- and ω6-fatty acids is of importance in several clinical situations. It has been demonstrated that the ω3-fatty acids are essential for the development of the retina and brain in premature children. Carlson and co-workers demonstrated the impact of feeding preterm infants with human breast milk and a formulation low in ω3-fatty acids (*figure 2*). The results revealed that the neonates given a formulation low in ω3-fatty acids exhibited decreased relative concentrations

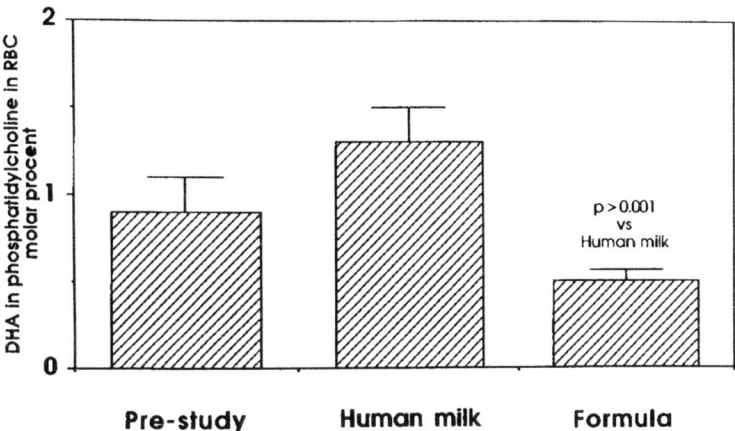

Figure 2. Docosahexaenoic acid status of preterm infants at birth and following feeding with human milk or formula (from [2]).

of docosahexaenoic acid in the phosphatidylcholine of their red blood cells. Even lower levels were found in brain after feeding newborn pigs a formulation low in ω3-fatty acids [3]. Neuringer [4] demonstrated that ω3-fatty acid deficient rhesus monkeys had subnormal visual activity at 4-12 weeks of age and prolonged recovery time of the dark adapted electroretinogram after a saturating flash. However, it remains to be defined whether dietary DHA may be as important to human infants for development of visual activity and cognitive learning as it apparently is to monkeys.

Another important aspect of the ω3-family of fatty acids is related to their impact on immune function and on the coagulation system. Mascioli and co-workers [5] demonstrated that animals subjected to endotoxin shock display an increased survival when fed on an ω3-fatty acid rich fish oil diet as compared to a diet based on safflower oil (figure 3). Endres with co-workers [6] showed recently that an ω3-fatty acid rich fish-oil diet fed to healthy volunteers suppressed the synthesis from monocytes of interleukin-1 and tumor necrosis factor, two cytokines with potent inflammatory capability. This suggests that the opportunity exists for manipulating the dietary composition of lipids as a pharmacological tool in order to influence the outcome of critical conditions associated with augmented inflammatory responses, as overactive immune system and endotoxic shock.

The ω3-fatty acids exert effects on the cardiovascular system which may be beneficial in some clinical situations where there is an augmented risk of arterial thrombosis and ischemia, e.g. heart surgery and myocardial infarction. The ω3-fatty acids induce a positive, antithrombotic balance between prostacyclines and thromboxanes [7]. Moreover, they possibly reduce the viscosity of whole blood [2] which may effectively improve the oxygen supply to tissues nourished by narrow vessels. An increase of the endogenous fibrinolytic activity has also been related to ω3-fatty acids; this by increasing the levels of tissue plasminogen activator and reducing the levels of inhibitors of plasminogen activator [9]. Finally, they increase

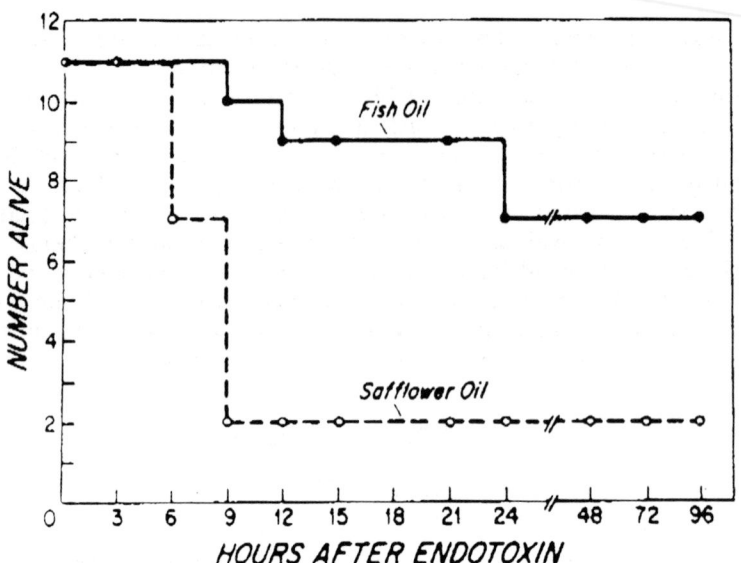

Figure 3. Survival curves of the two dietary groups. Curves differ by Kaplan-Meier analysis, p < 0.006 (from [5]).

the endothelial-dependent relaxation of coronary arteries in response to bradykinin, serotonin, adenosine diphosphate and thrombin [10].

Before ω3-fatty acids can be used as a pharmacological tool in new intravenous lipid emulsions, the dose needed to obtain the desired effects needs to be defined. Even more important possible adverse effects should be evaluated. The adverse effects which may be anticipated refer to lipid peroxidation, increased susceptibility to certain infections and prolongation of bleeding time [7]. Until now, none of these adverse effects have revealed substantial negative effects during clinical trials of oral fish-oil supplements.

MCT and structured lipids

The possibility to utilize medium-chain fatty acids (MCT) (C8 to C12) as an alternative energy source to the long-chain fatty acids has been the subject of significant interest over the last fifteen years. The rationale for the use of these fatty acids would be that they are a more readily available energy source than the LCT since they are only to a limited extent dependent on carnitine for transport into the mitochondria. In situations where carnitine may be limiting and the need for energy is high, e.g. in burn patients, MCT could be nitrogen-sparing.

Experimental data has indeed suggested that this can be the case. However, it is not yet demonstrated that an MCT/LCT physical mix emulsion can be administered during long-term TPN with the same safety features as an LCT containing lipid emulsion. Most regulatory authorities will not compromise on safety and tolerance even though certain metabolic advantages can be identified.

An alternative to a physical mix of MCT and LCT is that of an inter-esterified MCT/LCT containing triglyceride. Such triglycerides have been called structured triglycerides. The present structured lipid emulsions contain a random distribution of long and medium-chain fatty acids in the same triglyceride. Structured triglycerides have been evaluated in burned, septic and surgically stressed (partial hepatectomy) *(figure 4)* as well as animals sustained in cancer cachexia. In these catabolic situations, the emulsion has proven to have a nitrogen-sparing effect which is approximately 30% improved compared to that found with a traditional LCT containing lipid emulsion. This is concomitant with long-term tolerance studies demonstrating a similar tolerance to that found with LCT emulsions.

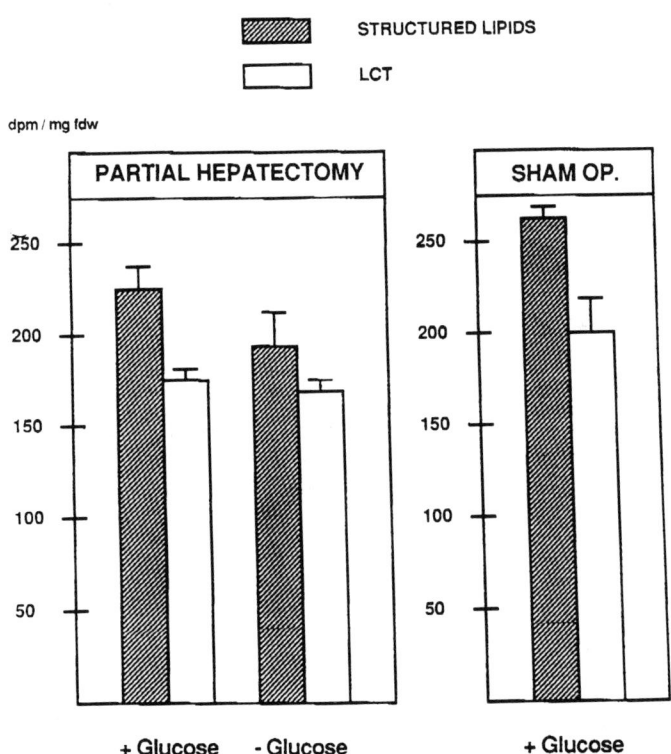

Figure 4. Effect of structured triglycerides on muscle protein systhesis in partially hepatectomized and sham-operated rats.

A reason for the discrepancy in tolerance between structured lipids and a physical mix of MCT/LCT may be related to a difference in the plasma kinetics of the medium-chain fatty acid. Preliminary data suggest that the pure MCT containing triglycerides are hydrolysed more rapidly than pure LCT containing triglycerides. However, when an emulsion with structured triglycerides is administered there is a random and slower efflux of medium-chain fatty acids into the plasma compartment as the triglycerides are hydrolysed.

Conclusion

When introducing new lipid emulsions to the medical community, one must distinguish between the scientific opportunity and the practical clinical reality. In order to achieve an acceptanbe from authorities as well as from clinicians, the new therapy has to be more effective and as safe as the current therapy. This in combination with the need for a more cost-effective therapy poses a challenge to industry as well as to the nutritionally oriented part of academia.

References

1. Friedman Z. Frohlich J.C. (1979) Essential fatty acids and the major urinary metabolites of the E prostaglandins in thriving neonates and in infants receiving parenteral fat emulsions. *Pediat. Res.* 13:932-935.
2. Carlson S.E., Rhodes P.G., Ferguson M.G. (1986) Docosahexaenoic acid status of preterm infants at birth and following feeding with human milk or formula. *Am. J. Clin. Nutr.* 44:798-804.
3. Innis S.M. (1988) Fats from terrestrial and marine animals and milk and tissue fatty acids in humans. NATO Advanced Research Workshop, Italy.
4. Neuringer M., Connor W.E., Lin D.S., Barstad L., Luck S. (1986) Biochemical and functional effects of prenatal and postnatal w3-fatty acid deficiency on retina and brain in rhesus monkeys. *Proc. Natl. Acad. Sci. USA* 43:4021-4025.
5. Mascioli E., Leader L., Flores E., Trimbo S., Bistrian B., Blackburn G. (1988) Enhanced survival to endotoxin in guinea pigs fed i.v. fish oil emulsion. *Lipids* 23:623-625.
6. Endres S., Ghorbani R., Kelley V. et al. 1989. The effect of dietary supplementation with n–3 polyunsaturated fatty acids on the synthesis of interleukin-1 and tumor necrosis factor by mononuclear cells. *N. Engl. J. Med.* 320:265-271.
7. Leaf A., Weber P.C. (1988) Cardiovascular effects of n–3 fatty acids. *N. Engl. J. Med.* 318:549-557.
8. Terano T., Hirai A., Hamazaki T. et al. (1983) Effect of oral administration of highly purified eicoapentaenoic acid on platelet function, blood viscosity and red cell deformability in healthy human subjects. *Atherosclerosis* 46, 321-331.
9. Barcelli U., Glas-Greenwalt P., Pollack V.E. (1985) Enhancing effect of dietary supplement with w3-fatty acids on plasma fibrinolysis in normal subjects. *Thromb. Res.* 39:307-312.
10. Shimokawa H., Lam J.Y.T., Chesebro J.H., Bowie E.J.W., Vanhoutte P.M. (1987) Effects of dietary supplementation with cod-liver oil on endothelium-dependent response in porcine coronary arteries. *Circulation* 76:898-905.

Summary

The safety and efficacy of present fat emulsions is well documented. Adult patients on long term fat emulsion treatment have not shown any tendency of essential acid deficiency syndrome. This indicates that the present emulsions do not only act as an energy source but also as a source of essential fatty acids (EFA). However in premature children EFA deficiency syndrome has been reported despite of an i.v. supply of fat emulsion.

Triglycerides from soy bean and safflower oil are presently used as a source of fatty acids. The majority of the essential fatty acids in these oils belong to the w6-series while w3-fatty acids are present in low amounts. EFAs are essential parts in all cell membranes and thereby a deficiency in EFAs will lead to various dysfunctions in cells and organs. These fatty acids have also a lipid lowering effect. Fatty acids belonging to the w3-series have been shown to be obligatory for the development of the retina and the brain in premature children while deficiency in fatty acids from the w6-series will lead to EFA deficiency syndromes. The inclusion of marine oils (rich in w3-fatty acids) in fat emulsions will decrease hyperlipidemia. Marine oils increase membrane fluidity, decrease blood viscosity and platelet aggregation. They have also been shown to increase the survival rate after endotoxic shock.

Premature children as well as elderly has decreased delta-6-desaturase activity, thus the formation of Y-linolenic acid and its products is decreased. This will result in EFA deficiency syndromes. A way to circumvent this blockate is to use oils rich in Y-linolenic acid. A balance between w3- and w6-fatty acids will improve the effect of fat emulsions both in the body's normal physiological state and in specific therapeutic conditions. Fatty acids from the w6-series are the precursors for the most potent prostanoids, which in case of overproduction may result in deleterious effects. Fatty acids from the w3-series are known to antagonize such an over-production.

Further implication of this will be a direction of specific fatty acids to specific targets. This could theoretically be achieved by a selective incorporation of the fatty acids into a triglyceride molecule (structured lipids).

The above improvements concomitantly with an improved stability and compatibility can be foreseen for emulsions of the nineties.

Discussion

Dr Martinez: I don't know anything about the practical problems from the pharmaceutical point of view, but don't you think it would be better to add some more physiological phospholipid than just a fish oil. I'm a little concerned about this problem because the very high content of fish oils in EPA; perhaps this is too much, you cannot find any tissue in the human body with this high content of EPA. Perhaps it would be much more physiological to have, if it is technically possible I don't know, some phosphatidylserine for example.

Dr Ekman: Well, for one thing I think that it is possible to manipulate the relation, but the amount that EPA versus DHA in fish oils, that technically possible to do, to do the step that you suggested is probably also possible to do but the cost would be very high. We have to remember that we deal with a nutrient which is already relatively expensive for the end user. If the end user, that is the patient or the physician has to pay that increased amount of money we have to prove a significant efficacy. But if we can do so, yes it's possible.

Dr Bjerve: I think the way you presented the talk was very interesting and I think it is very important to work along the lines you mentioned not to use biochemical parameters, be it fatty acid composition in tissues and cells and organs, whatever, I think we will have to deal with rate of complications, rate of success in treatment, rate of weight gain and positive nitrogen balance and things like that. I think we will have to work on those lines when we are trying to make the final fatty acid composition. We can speculate from a lot of standpoints, is it bad or good to have much EPA, is it bad or good to have much DHA, can we use gamma linolenic or not. The ultimate answer lies in experiments, testing these hypothesis.

Dr Ekman: I agree.

Chairman: A question,

Dr Messing: It's just a comment concerning the possibility of interest of giving gammalinolenic in ulcerative colitis you mentioned in one of your slides. I'm not sure that for the adult population that this is a good goal because now it has been established that for severe flare up of ulcerative colitis the best choice is to give the patients to the surgeon. But I think that in certain circumstances you can need a TPN for ulcerative colitis for example, post operative complications, but since you mentioned prostaglandin possibility or anti-inflammatory effect of such a product I think it could be better to replace in your slide ulcerative colitis by crohn disease.

Dr Ekman: Thank you for your comment. This slide was constructed after the literature by addressing the reports where you have a decreased activity of delta 6 desaturase, I think we are way away from talking of efficacy, I also stated that personally I believe with what I know that only opportunity would be in the infants to prove any kind of efficacy so I agree.

Chairman: I have the same question for the cystic fibrosis that you mentioned and about the ability of gammalinolenic acid and I would ask about the problem of peroxidation because in this patient there is very frequently a very low vitamin E status.

Dr Ekman: On the same token this was up on the list because there had been proven to be low in delta 6 desaturase. I think, however, that the interest in this patient group is significant because we have received a number of requests from physicians worldwide treating their patient group who want to test the hypothesis. I do acknowledge the peroxidation problem and that has to be addressed before we can do anything, I think it's possible to solve it.

Pr Bach: We measured lipoprotein lipase and hepatic lipase activity on structured lipids and we observed that the activity was a bit slower *with structured lipids and with MCT but was much more quick than for LCT.*

Dr Ekman: Exactly; that actually is excellent support for our kinetic data, that the relative appearance of the MCT in this setting is in between that of the MCT where it flushes south into the vascular system as compared to the slower release of the LCTs. So that fits very well to the in vivo data.

Dr Friedman: I really enjoyed your excellent presentation, I just have one question, can you elaborate about the addition of carnitine for intralipid for low birth weight infants.

Dr Ekman: I believe that the question is very pertinent because if you have, if you look at the carnitine level in colostrum it's certainly high, and we also know that the pre-term infants cannot synthesize carnitine at the needed level. So in the carnitine field doing the same kind of analyses I believe that this specific patient group there is an opportunity to prove efficacy by adding carnitine to let's say an intralipid formula. I think there is in this a selected situation.

Dr Adam: I should like to ask whether the improved protein synthesis with other structure lipids was related to a better energy supply or was just related to maybe some structural improvements in the cells.

Dr Ekman: Well, all animals received an identical amount of energy and it was controlled for the amount of nitrogen energy, trace elements and so on; so that cannot be the explanation. I do not know exactly why the structured lipid could retain more nitrogen in this situation. From the speculative point of view, I would believe that the requirements for energy substrates are higher in the mitochondria, maybe carnitine could be limiting or maybe the combination of the usage of LCT and MCT in this situation could be an advantage. This observation has also been seen in MCT–LCT combination that there is an improvement of the nitrogen retention, however it's more pronounced, this may be related to the fact that the cell gets to see the MCT over a longer period of time.

Pr Bach: I have been told about the emulsion used to slow down the development of tumors and I have been told that some fatty acids act better than some others. May I ask you which fatty acids are used in these structured lipids.

Dr Ekman: The objective here is not to cure cancer. This was a group of investigators who are interested to use the structured lipids in order to increase the nitrogen retention in the carcass of the host; but it was more an accidental finding, the design of the study was not really to address what it did to the tumor. I don't think nutrition can cure cancer, I think we have to remember that nutrition is only used as an adjunct to help the patient survive the treatment and after spending ten years in the field of cancer and nutrition, I believe that the opportunities are limited to manipulate our nutrients in order to make tumor growth lower or quicker, because we can manipulate that in the clinical practice by other means, by taking away the tumor or radiate it or give it cytostatic drugs, the important is to feed the host so it can survive the treatment.

Dr Friedman: One of the concerns that some of the participants has about intralipid is the excessive amount of linoleic acid. Did you consider to reduce the amount of linoleic acid and substitute it with just other monosaturate or saturated fatty acids for caloric substrate.

Dr Ekman: I believe that by introducing new oil combinations you will decrease the relative amount of linoleic acid. I think it would be extremely costly to go in and let's say chop out part of any fatty acid, it would be a costly procedure. And in the very cost containment situation we are today I don't think we as physicians would like to pay a significantly larger price for such a product if we cannot prove that it makes a very big difference. That's a sort of a very Harvard answer because it didn't really address what you said, but I think the cost issue here is really critical.

Chairman: Any more questions. So perhaps you want to have some general discussion or we consider we stop now. I think I can speak for all the participants to thank again all the people taking part there, orators, organisors, Prof Ghisolfi and Kabivitrume team.

Photocomposition et impression
IMPRIMERIE LOUIS-JEAN
BP 87 — 05003 GAP Cedex
Tél. : 92.51.35.23
Dépôt légal : 492 — Juillet 1990
Imprimé en France